Selene Yeager's
Perfectly
Fit™

Selene Yeager's
Perfectly Fit™

8 Weeks
to a Sleek and Sexy Body

By **SELENE YEAGER** Strength Trainer, Mountain Bike Racer,
Fitness Consultant, Columnist, Author, *Bicycling* Magazine's Fitness Chick

RODALE®

Printed in the United States of America
Rodale Inc. makes every effort to use acid-free ∞, recycled paper ♻.

Interior Designer: Joanna Williams
Cover Designer: Christopher Rhoads
Interior Photographs: Mitch Mandel/Rodale Images

Library of Congress Cataloging-in-Publication Data
Yeager, Selene.
   Selene Yeager's perfectly fit : 8 weeks to a sleek and sexy body / by Selene Yeager.
       p.   cm.
   Includes index.
   ISBN 1–57954–410–X hardcover
   ISBN 1–57954–316–2 paperback
   1. Exercise for women.   2. Physical fitness for women.   3. Weight training for women.
   I. Title: Perfectly fit.   II. Title.
   GV482 .Y43   2001
   613.7'045—dc21   00–067338

Distributed to the book trade by St. Martin's Press

2 4 6 8 10 9 7 5 3 1   hardcover
2 4 6 8 10 9 7 5 3 1   paperback

Visit us on the Web at www.rodalesportsandfitness.com, or call us toll-free at (800) 848-4735.

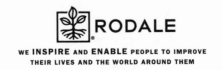

WE **INSPIRE** AND **ENABLE** PEOPLE TO IMPROVE
THEIR LIVES AND THE WORLD AROUND THEM

contents

Part 5
Perfectly Fit: The Attitude

salvation in strength training

It's easier than you think to get the body you want

have always been a big girl. As far back as second grade, I remember our pediatrician handing my mom my first diet. It didn't work; diets never do. Although I was active in school sports like field hockey and track, I still tipped the scales at 150 pounds by high school and had to buy bigger clothes every school year, even though I should have long since stopped being a growing girl.

So, like any stupid high school girl, I started smoking. That was only marginally helpful. And, of course, it was really great for my sports performance. The stupidity worsened once I got to college. Terrified of adding the "freshman 15" to my already well-padded frame, I started starving myself. I'll spare you the dirty details, but after almost 2 years of anorexic behavior, I weighed 105 pounds and looked like hell, as my hair literally began to fall out, my skin dried and cracked, and my mother threatened to admit me to the hospital.

Somehow, I pulled through. I started eating "normally" again, did a little jogging, and took some aerobics classes. But still, slowly and surely, my weight crept back up to almost 150, and I was miserable about it. Not only because I didn't like the way the weight made me look but also because I really hated the way it made me feel. I hated the sluggishness, the way it sapped my energy, and the way it prevented me from physically enjoying life to the fullest. For a while, I tried body-building, but all of those bulk-building sets and reps only weighed me down more.

Finally, I started some sensible strength training: moderate sets, higher reps, and integrated total-body exercises. Over the course of a couple of years, I dropped four dress sizes. I discovered my love for sports again and started competing in mountain bike races and triathlons. Within my first couple of years in the sport, I found that I had the fitness and strength to win some medals and even qualified for the world championship race in X-terra, an off-road triathlon series. I figured that if these exercise philosophies could help transform me from a chunky smoker to a strong amateur athlete, they could help millions of women.

So I got serious about studying physiology and became certified as a trainer. I started training women and men one on one, began teaching group exercise classes, and started sharing ways to get fit as a journalist working for *Bicycling*, *Prevention*, *Men's Health*, *Fitness*, and other magazines. In short, fitness became my calling. And I finally stopped worrying about my weight.

Every Woman's Story

I write this because I know that millions of women suffer through similar struggles. I meet them every day in the programs I run and in the classes I teach. They've tried every diet. They've taken every supplement. They've jumped on every exercise craze. Yet they are still literally weighed down by excess bulk that saps their energy, lowers their confidence, and makes them less likely to engage life in any physical way. What's worse, studies show that being overweight often prevents women from enjoying a healthy, active sex life. So their relationships suffer as well.

Time and time again, these women are amazed at the body-transforming power of strength training. The science of it is simple: Strength training builds muscle. Muscle takes up about half the space of fat and is more metabolically active. Each pound of muscle burns up to 50 calories a day just maintaining itself. Each pound of fat burns just 2 calories. Lift weights a few times a week and you'll build muscle and burn fat. Even though your actual weight won't decrease as much as you may expect, because muscle tissue is heavier than fat, you'll lose inches and feel lighter because you're stronger.

And that's just the tip of the transformation. Strong, toned muscles do more than give you a tight body in a sundress. When you are fit and strong, you feel more confident. And when you feel more confident, you're more willing to take some risks in life. Lifting weights gave me the body confidence to take up cycling, running, and swimming, and eventually to start racing. Competing gave me the confidence to start my own business. And so on. I've seen women in their fifties start riding bikes again, sign up to learn new sports like sea kayaking, and literally walk 2 inches taller—all because they picked up some weights and discovered they could. I've seen insecure women in their twenties and thirties finally stand up to pushy boyfriends and demeaning bosses after making a little muscle of their own.

The fact is, women of all sizes and ages simply exude a sexy "I can" attitude after they start strength training. And why not? With their new-found strength, they're no longer shackled to a bad body image. They're burning tons more calories every day, so they don't have to fret over every morsel that goes into their mouths. They're physically stronger, so they can carry heavy packages, move furniture, and open jars without any assistance. And they look and feel younger, fitter, and more energetic than they have in years—maybe in their entire lives.

That's my wish for every woman who picks up this book. May you get the body you've always wanted and do everything you've ever dreamed. Now rock on. And get started.

PART 1

PERFECTLY FIT

FIT

the foundation

what is perfectly fit?

Strong muscles and sexy tone wrapped in a can-do attitude

When I first started strength training, I was dating an Arnold Schwarzenegger disciple who was gung ho to introduce me to the world of bodybuilding. We would grunt and hoist massive weights, performing three or four exercises and countless reps and sets on every single little muscle in a vain—literally!—search for the ultimate pump. After 6 months of that joyless exercise, my biceps were bulging, my calves were curving, and I could crack walnuts on my ass (well . . . almost).

But God forbid I actually had to swing a racket, run a 5-K, or ski down a hill. I had overly developed somewhat impressive but practically useless muscles. Plus, they weren't "all that" in the appearance category, either. Through all those hours of lifting, I had bulked up and looked and felt awkward and unbalanced.

A little discouraged, I scaled back on the endless exercises and repetitions. I included more fluid moves that I learned and sometimes adapted from yoga, athlete training centers, and simple strengthening and toning classes. I lost the bulk, improved the tone, and got fit enough to start competing in recreational cycling and running.

That's when it really came together.

Once I began competing, I started studying methods for working my muscles in more integrated ways, like how I used them in real life. There, I found medicine balls, compound-combination moves, core-body exercises, and much more. I started creating and stringing exercises together in total-body programs. And before I knew it, I had muscle tone that not only looked better than ever but also performed better. No, I could no longer win free beer in arm-wrestling contests, but when I hit the trails or sliced through the water, my muscles harmonized together like a well-rehearsed symphony. The sweetest part: These exercises maintained my strength and tone even when I wasn't competing.

Bursting with enthusiasm, I started sharing these exercises with clients. Even women and men who had religiously pumped iron for years couldn't believe the transformation. Abs firmed, butts lifted, and love handles disappeared.

Sexy and Seamless

Because these exercises challenge and strengthen many muscles at the same time—the way you use them in life—they vastly improve how gracefully and balanced you hold yourself and how nimbly you move through everyday tasks. Because they emphasize total-body toning including core, major, and supporting muscles, your entire physique will streamline. Instead of having fab abs or killer legs on a so-so body, you'll have seamless tone from head to heels.

That said, you'll quickly notice that not every exercise in this book is a multimuscle integrated move. It's important to start with a solid founda-tion. And because we tend to overuse some muscles and totally neglect others, many women have muscle imbalances. That's why I start newcomers off with a mix of traditional isolation exercises (one muscle group at a time) along with just a few easy combination moves. As they build a strong overall foundation, we use those muscles together with more challenging, integrated exercises. As the programs progress, there are fewer (though more challenging) isolation exercises and more Perfectly Fit combination moves to fully develop strength, tone, posture, and balance.

The Stuff You'll Need

As you flip through the book, you'll see training equipment of all shapes and sizes. There are balls, bands, body weights, and dumbbells. It looks like a hell of an investment, but don't be scared off. You can buy everything you need to do this program for less than $100. And even if you own just a pair of dumbbells right now, you can still get started. Though medicine balls are ideal for many of the core body moves, a single dumbbell will often work well in a pinch. You'll notice that I've indicated the exercises that allow for easy equipment substitutions.

So why all the different stuff? It's not because I'm a gearhead or have stock in equipment manufacturers. It's just that, in keeping with the Perfectly Fit philosophy, the more ways you can work your muscles, the better developed they'll be, and the more toned you'll become. All of these instruments offer different forms of resistance for your body, so your muscles will never feel stale and your mind will never get bored.

I also want you to go above and beyond the programs you find here. There are more than 80 exercises total and a chapter on DIY (Do-It-Yourself) Programming to put you on the road to creating your own programs once you feel ready to do it. There are also tons of workout ideas included in chapter 5, which explains the many modalities for strength training. Dig in and go nuts.

Be a Go-To Girl

I encourage you time and again to take your strong, agile body out into the world and do something with it. Part of the Perfectly Fit philosophy is that your body was meant to move. It gets more beautiful and youthful the more you use it to dance, play, and run. Engage life large. Don't ever be afraid of failing or making a fool of your-self. Quite the contrary, those around you will admire your spirit for trying.

The back section of this book offers a large variety of activities for you to sample. None of them is extreme; all are healthy, accessible sports and active hobbies that will further shape your body, challenge your mind, and enliven your spirit. Sitting on our butts 24/7 is a very modern development. And it's killing us . . . literally. Refuse to live a sedentary life. You'll be happier, healthier, and, of course, more fit.

Think you don't have time? Perfectly Fit women make the time. They and their active lives, as well as the active lives of their families, are *the* priority. If that concept is a struggle, scope the advice in part 5.

Then take that one beautiful body you have and go conquer this one life you've been given to live. All you have to do is try.

strong, lean, and happy

Why every woman must strength train

Maybe, like so many women, you sometimes wonder why you should even bother with strength training. Or maybe it's one of those things you know you *should* do, but never get around to. Well, if you're serious about ditching the flab and unveiling a beach-ready bod, strength training is the only way.

That's right, the only way. For years, however, women were sold the same bill of goods: If you want to burn fat, be fit, and achieve body Nirvana, aerobics is the answer. And each year, millions of leotard-clad women poured into aerobic dance classes hoping to look like the babes in the health club ads, only to come out with bodies that looked startlingly similar to the ones they started with. I saw this happen time and again among women in the classes I taught, and I saw it in myself, too.

Don't get me wrong: We were a whole lot healthier from the workouts. All that cardiovascular activity blasts stress and builds healthier hearts and lungs. And it definitely burns extra calories. But when you're looking for total body toning—you know, the stuff we all like to have, like lean legs and shapely arms—aerobics alone just doesn't do the job.

But strength training does because it doesn't just burn calories while you do it.

It increases your muscle mass, which helps you burn more calories all day long. What's more, strength training gives you great curves, super posture, better bones, and even provides a lot of the same benefits as aerobic exercise.

A woman I've trained with, marathon runner and editor Alisa Bauman, age 30, says it best: "I run, cycle, do yoga, swim, play sports, and eat well, but all the dieting and aerobic exercise in the world doesn't give me the type of body I can get from lifting weights." The problem is, even though many women today have heard all about the wonders of weight training, many still haven't given it a try. As one client said when asked why she waited so long to start lifting, "I just never believed it could make that big of a difference."

As you will soon see, it really can.

Metabolism Magic

In a nutshell, strength training works because making muscles fires up your metabolism and keeps your body running at its fat-burning best. (This is why many men can toss down a bucket of wings and a pitcher of beer without a worry about weight gain—they naturally have more muscle.) Every pound of muscle on your body burns between 30 and 50 calories a day—even when you're sleeping. Every pound of fat burns only 2 to 5 calories. Women often blame their weight problems on sluggish metabolisms when what's really to blame is their lack of muscle.

Unless you start strength training, the problem only gets worse. As we get older, we naturally lose some of our muscle mass. Starting somewhere

after age 35, women start losing about a half-pound of muscle a year. By age 50, that can jump to up to a pound loss each year. That's why women in their late thirties and forties often complain that even though they are not eating or exercising differently, they are still gaining weight—they are literally losing metabolism-revving muscle. Obviously, the more sedentary you are, the worse this scenario becomes.

The great news is that you can stop this early midlife fat spread in its tracks just by adding a little muscle. Researchers at Tufts University in Medford, Massachusetts, found that people who strength trained for 12 weeks and increased their muscle mass by just 3 pounds could eat 15 percent more calories—that's about 300 calories (the amount in two slices of cheese pizza!) a day for an average woman—without gaining an ounce. Even better, they also lost fat pounds in the process.

Over time, these muscle-metabolism gains can add up to major fat losses. Consider this: If you gain 3 pounds of muscle and burn 40 additional calories per pound, you'll burn 120 additional calories per day, or 3,600 calories per month. At that rate, those 3 pounds of muscle will burn off 12 pounds over the course of a year.

"When I started weight training, I saw results within 3 weeks. My pants became loose around the waist. I could see my arms toning up. I just looked better in the same clothes, even though I was technically 'gaining weight,'" recalls editor Bridget Doherty, 29. "That never happened with any other exercise before."

Strength-training researchers have studied this effect on thousands of women, and the results are remarkable, no matter at what age the study participants began.

Compact Powerhouse

Adding muscle tissue will also make you stronger yet more compact, so you'll feel like a lean, yet powerful, woman. But be aware: That means tossing out your conventional ideas about "weight" and judging your progress by how you look, feel, and perform instead.

The easiest way to understand the dynamics of strength training is to remember these two cardinal rules. One: Muscle tissue takes up considerably less space (and is much more aesthetically pleasing) than fat tissue. Two: Muscle tissue weighs more than fat tissue. Too often, women who are having fabulous success with their fitness programs step on a scale and get discouraged because they haven't lost as much weight as they hoped to. Their clothes fit better. They feel better. They look great. But they're still sweating the numbers on the scale.

Your better bet is to pay attention to your measurements. Is your waistline getting trimmer? Are your legs firmer? Do your clothes hang better? You can also get your body composition tested at your local health club. Or test it yourself with a home monitoring device—Tanita and Body Logic both make good home-testing models. Body composition testing gives you a better picture of what's actually happening as you lose body fat and gain strength, because it breaks your weight into lean tissue and fat tissue. And it's highly motivating to see those numbers change.

By monitoring your clothes, appearance, and

between YOU&ME

Like many women today, I never knew body confidence until I started strength training. Just hated shorts. Avoided pools and beaches. Didn't even like people watching me walk. There is no greater freedom than slipping on some hip shorts and heading downtown without once stressing about your legs or your butt. There is no greater high than actually using those strong legs and buns to climb a mountain or surf a wave. It's not about being skinny. It's about being strong.

body composition, you also can ditch any fears you might have about "bulking up." Some women still worry that strength training will make them bigger instead of trimmer. While it may give you more noticeable muscles in certain areas, like shapely, round shoulders and beautiful, curvy biceps, it will help you tighten, tone, and get more lean overall because muscle raises your metabolism, helps you burn fat, and, again, takes up less space than fat. Plus, women simply don't have the hormones necessary to bulk up à la Sly Stallone through simple strength training. It takes hours of lifting, and usually a little outside stimulus, for females to build real bulk. In fact, exercise scientists have found that women can build lean tissue and improve their upper-body strength by 40 percent without seeing real changes in body size. Through moderate weight training—that's two or three times a week—you can expect to increase your strength by 30 to 50 percent. Get the picture?

"Lifting weights has started to slim me down in areas that wouldn't benefit this early in a cardio-only program. And I love the feeling when I'm done, like I'm becoming a finely tuned machine," says Lisa Neyen, 35, a software engineer and mother of two.

The Skeleton Key

We all know that women are at an increased risk for osteoporosis. Since we can't see our bones, it's a totally out of sight, out of mind threat for most young women. But just take one look at some frail, elderly women in your neighborhood and it shouldn't take you long to realize that you don't want to end up shuffling and hunched over one day. Again, strength training is key.

Once you've reached adulthood, you've basically made your bones as dense as they'll ever be. Past that point, and especially once you near menopause, your bones begin to lose calcium and other minerals, which can make them more porous and likely to break, unless you take protective measures to keep building them back up.

The National Osteoporosis Foundation recommends that you get 1,000 to 1,500 milligrams of calcium a day—take a supplement to be sure. Walking, running, and other weight-bearing aerobic exercise can help build your lower-body bones. But the best way to keep all your bones solid and dense is strength training. Research shows that just 6 months of weight training can increase spinal bone mineral density by up to 13 percent.

Strong bones will also help you hold on to your height as you get older. Ever notice how women seem to shrink as they get older? That's because their vertebrae become brittle and actually begin to compress. This is what leads to the hunchbacked appearance common among older women in the pre–strength training generations. Unless you're eager to follow in their frail footsteps, pick up some weights and get moving.

Live Longer and Happier

For the longest time, aerobic exercise got all of the accolades for fending off chronic ailments like diabetes and heart disease. But now scientists believe that time in the weight room may be just as beneficial as hours in aerobics class for preventing disease. Studies show that weight training can lower cholesterol levels, blood pressure, and body fat—all important factors in the fight to keep your heart healthy. The American Heart Association Science Advisory now recommends strength training 2 or 3 days a week.

Strength training also improves glucose metabolism. That means your body will be better able to process insulin and regulate your blood sugar, so you'll be less likely to succumb to adult-onset diabetes—a growing problem for both men and women as our nation's waistline grows ever wider. Research shows that just 4 months of weight training can increase your glucose metabolism by 23 percent. That's powerful protection.

Maybe best of all, strength training can make you happy. For one, strength training is a great way to blow out the stress, anxiety, and tension of the day. You'll sleep like a stone at night, as your body demands high-quality sleep to recover from your workouts. Studies show that you'll be less likely to suffer from depression, an ailment that clouds women's lives more often than men's. And you'll simply feel good about yourself. Strong, toned muscles make women ooze confidence and live comfortably in their bodies like nothing else I've seen.

"My strength training has helped me look and feel stronger, which I equate with feeling more beautiful, capable, and confident," says Liz Reap, 31, a photographer and Fuji team-sponsored cyclist. "My posture has improved, my attitude about myself has improved, and I feel more balanced."

Play More and Better

If you play sports, strength training will make you play better. If you don't play sports, strength training will make you want to go out and play.

When your muscles are strong, you can run faster, cycle better, throw farther, and swing a racket with more power. You're less likely to get hurt because strong muscles support your joints while you play, helping you avoid sprains and strains. You have better balance, making you more sure on your feet. Even better, you can recover from tough exertion more quickly. "I've seen a remarkable improvement on the bike since I started strength training," says Reap. "I have more muscle endurance and pure power. I don't fatigue as quickly. And I recover better, so I don't have lingering soreness for days after a tough race."

Even women who tend to shy away from sports find themselves becoming more physically active once they pick up weight training. "Because I saw such a difference in myself with strength training, I was encouraged to try more," says Doherty. "Without planning on it, I noticed that I started to walk more and try activities that I wouldn't have tried before."

These benefits are especially pronounced for women who are currently out of shape or overweight. The fact is, even though physical activity is what they need most, many overweight women avoid exercise like oral surgery—and not unreasonably so. Frankly, exercise can really suck when you're out of shape. It's no fun feeling winded and sore doing something that's supposed to make you feel so spectacular. Weight training is less intimidating and more accessible than running or even walking when you're out of shape or overweight. Then, once those muscles get a little stronger, walking around the block isn't such a big deal. You start becoming more spontaneously active simply because you feel more capable and confident.

"The exercises were so simple, I wasn't sure they would make any difference when I started," says Jodya Wasilko, 57, a client of mine who, frustrated by many years of feeling unfit, started strength training 2 years ago. "But soon, daily activities became so much easier. I was redecorating my house and moving furniture like it was nothing. I even signed up for my first charity walk. It was a great accomplishment."

accessorize yourself

What to wear, what to try, what to buy

A sk the salesperson at your local sporting goods store what you need to start weight training and you're sure to walk out with a whole lot more than you'll use. After an initial small investment in a few weights and maybe a mat and a step or bench, there's not much more you need. But there's tons more you *could* buy. A high-energy sales rep may try to sell you on hand wraps, waist belts, knee braces, even special socks. Don't immediately buy into it. Most of it is unnecessary.

Here's a no-nonsense guide to what you need—and what you don't—in the wide world of workout gear.

Clothes: Form and Function

You could lift weights butt naked if you wanted. But wearing the right attire can make it a whole lot easier, more effective, and probably safer. You'll be happiest if you wear clothes that are stretchy enough to let you reach and bend freely without restricting your range of motion. Here's what to look for.

Form-fitting. Like millions of women, you'll likely be tempted to toss on the standard camouflage workout uniform: A pair of leggings and an oversize T-shirt. Resist the urge. I know it covers up every little bulge, but that's the problem—it covers up every little bulge, including your muscles. You want to be able to see that your back is straight, your shoulders are down, and the proper muscles are working during your routine. Since you're at home, you need not be self-conscious. Opt for a tank top and tights (or baggy pants if you prefer), so you can see your torso. The hidden benefit: You'll be able to watch your muscle tone improve.

Breathable fabric. Cotton is great for picnics and lounging. But if you're going to be exercising and breaking a light sweat, one of today's new synthetic moisture-wicking fabrics such as Dri-Fit is the way to go. Cotton gets damp, stays damp, and leaves you chilled, but these fabrics pull moisture away from your body, leaving you warm and comfy.

Supportive. Since you won't be jumping around, you can get away with lifting in a regular, supportive bra. But you'll definitely be more comfortable in a sports bra. Sports bras were designed to move in, so they're less likely to ride up, pinch, or bind. You can even buy ones that zip up the front, so they're super-easy to put on and take off.

Attractive. Do yourself a favor and pick up an attractive workout outfit. I don't care if you're just a few pounds overweight or 50 pounds, how you dress has a big influence on how you feel. If you have a great outfit, you'll be more eager to put it on and get moving. And when you feel sharp and sexy, you stand a little taller and put a little more energy into your activity than when you feel dumpy and unattractive.

Shoes: Your Sole Support

I've seen people weight train in everything from thong sandals to penny loafers. Sure, any shoes will protect the soles of your feet, but everyday shoes don't offer much support for the rest of your body. If you really want, you can buy special weight lifting shoes (there truly is a shoe for everything), but that's not necessary. Simply look for a pair of athletic shoes with the following qualities. If you already have them, you're good to go.

Ankle support. Many moves in the Perfectly Fit System require a fair amount of balance. As you lunge forward and back and side to side, a good pair of shoes can help keep you stable. Look for shoes that are cut a little higher around the ankle (you don't need high-tops, however) and that feel supportive when you step from side to side.

Flexibility. Some exercises have you up on the balls of your feet. These moves are easier to do if you have some flexibility in the arch of your shoe. Hold your shoe in both hands with one hand on the heel and one around the toebox area, and try to bend it. If the sole has some play in it, you'll be fine. If it's seriously difficult to budge the sole back and forth, you might consider finding a more flexible pair.

Fit. Women are notorious for stuffing their feet into shoes that don't fit. I once ran a half-marathon in shoes a half-size too small! You need a solid, comfortable base when you strength train. That means shoes that let your toes spread into

between
YOU&ME

their natural position and don't cramp your feet. And remember: Your feet can grow throughout adulthood—especially if you've been pregnant. If those old size 7s don't fit like they used to, get measured for a new pair.

Gloves and Wraps: A Second Skin

Gloves used to be a must-have in the weight room—mostly because they were a fashion statement. Now you rarely see them. I've tried weight training both ways, and I've ditched the gloves, mainly because it's one less thing I have to think about and they didn't offer much assistance anyway. Ditto for hand wraps, the more macho (and complicated) alternative to gloves.

One exception: If you have very small hands or sensitive skin, gloves might give you a boost. Most weight-lifting gloves are padded across the upper palm, right below your finger line, so they reduce some of the pressure of the weights. They also protect your skin from the sometimes rough metal bars on dumbbells, so you'll be less likely to develop calluses, if that is a concern.

Belts and Braces: Use Sparingly

Weight-lifting belts may look cool, but you won't be needing one for the Perfectly Fit System. In fact, they can actually be counterproductive in this program. As you may recall from seeing them on gargantuan power-lifters, weight-lifting belts are wide, thick belts that cover your lower back and buckle in the front over your abdomen. The theory is that they're supposed to support your lower back while you lift. In reality, though they can offer some support during *very* heavy squats and overhead presses, studies show that they are of little use for most lifters. What's more, if you do all your strength training with a weight belt on, you won't fully develop your supporting back and abdominal muscles, which is one of the reasons you're working out. By keeping your abdominal muscles tight, you can get all the support you need, and you'll develop nice tight abs in the process.

In the same vein as belts are knee and elbow braces. Usually made of constrictive Neoprene, these braces fit over your joints to support them while you lift. Again, a major point of strength training is building the muscles and connective tissues around these joints, which you won't do if you're relying on a brace. As a general rule: If you need a brace, you're lifting too much weight.

Bottles and Towels: Nice Touches

My water bottle is a permanent fixture in my gym bag. Where I go, it goes. Though you obviously don't need a water bottle to work out, I recommend it. A plastic water bottle is cheap and portable, so you can throw it into a suitcase when you're working out on the road. And because they come equipped with squeeze-squirt tops, you won't spill water all over the floor if you knock it over while exercising. Having your water bottle handy also reminds you to stay hydrated while you work out—a good idea even if you aren't sweating, because it keeps you cool and energized.

A little workout towel is a nice touch. If you're quick to break a sweat (and don't fancy wiping your brow with your shirt), keep one handy by your water bottle.

Log Book: Keeping It Real

Studies show that dieters who keep food journals are more successful at losing weight than those who don't. I believe the same is true for exercisers. When you write something down, it makes it real. It also makes it easier to remember. I keep a little journal where I record the exercises I did, how much weight, the number of sets and reps. It's nice to leaf through the journal once in a while and take pride in the progress I've made. I'm also less likely to blow off exercises when I have them down in black and white!

You'll find a sample journal page on page 191, and there are blank journal pages starting on page 277. Feel free to make copies of these and keep them in a three-ring binder for record-keeping.

the basics and beyond

What you need to know about lifting weights

t's about as basic as it gets. You raise the weight, then you lower the weight. Yet strength training can be confusing even for experienced lifters. Little decisions like how much weight to use, what muscles to work, and how many sets and reps to do all add up to big differences in the kind of results you'll achieve. I think every woman should know the scientific "why" behind what she's doing. It's part of working that beautiful brain along with those biceps. Also, by understanding the theory behind strength-training principles, you'll be able to develop your own programs down the road as well as tailor any plan to fit your specific likes and needs.

Getting Started

When you have a busy schedule and an hour to exercise, the urge to dive right in is strong. Resist. Instead, take 5 to 10 minutes to jump rope, ride a Spinning bike, or jog up and down off a step. This brief warmup increases your body temperature and warms your muscles, making them more supple and receptive, so you're less likely to suffer a pull or a strain. Warming up also makes your workouts work better by priming all of your energy systems.

Here are the benefits of just 10 minutes of moving your muscles.

❐ Boosts delivery of oxygen and fuel to muscles, so they're better prepared for strenuous tasks

❐ Opens pores and brings you to a light sweat, so your body is primed to keep itself cool and you're less likely get red-faced and overheated

❐ Activates the production of important enzymes in your body's energy system, so you're more efficient at turning stored fuel into energy and you won't end up feeling prematurely fatigued

❐ Speeds up the transmission of nerve impulses, which improves your coordination and helps you perform your exercises with greater skill

So I don't care if you're a marathoner or a reformed channel surfer, a warmup is essential for everybody.

Pick the Right Weight

To make stronger, more toned muscles, you need to challenge your muscle fibers. You can't do that unless you lift a weight that is challenging. Too many women don't get the results they want because they're lifting a weight that is lighter than your typical romance novel. Generally speaking, the weight you choose should be heavy enough so that the last 4 repetitions are tough, and you absolutely can't lift beyond 12 to 15. Though many fitness magazines show sexy, shapely, kick-ass women holding tiny 2-pound dumbbells, that weight is not sufficient for women who regularly heft heavier items while making dinner. And those models didn't make those muscles lifting those weights.

Once you reach the point where you can easily perform all of the repetitions with strength to spare—and that happens quickly with beginning lifters—it's time to increase your weight to keep your muscles challenged. Simply move up to the next closest weight (from 8 pounds to 10 pounds, for example). Or you can use magnetic Plate-Mates. These are small, flat weights that you can stick on the ends of dumbbells to increase the weight in 1- to 3-pound increments. They're perfect when you have dumbbells that increase on a 5-pound scale, which can be too big of a jump. Also, whenever you increase your weight, you can lower your number of reps (from 15 to 10, for example) until your strength improves.

Order Your Exercise

The Perfectly Fit System orders your routines so you perform exercises that emphasize your big muscles, like your gluteus (glutes for short), back, and chest, before those that challenge your smallest muscles like your arms and shoulders. This is a standard fitness rule, because those small muscles need to be fresh and strong to support your big muscles through challenging moves like squats, lunges, and chest presses. Once they've performed those important duties, then you can fatigue them with their own exercises. A whole-body sequence would be glutes, legs, back, arms, and shoulders.

Some people (especially bodybuilders) recommend "split" routines, where instead of working through your whole body, you work some muscles (like chest, back, and arms) on some days and other muscles (legs, glutes) on other days. The advantage here is that you can devote more time to doing more exercises for each muscle group, which works well for bodybuilders who routinely perform five separate arm curls to develop their biceps to ridiculous proportions. And it's okay if you like to lift 4 or 5 days a week. But it's not necessary for most women, and it's overdoing it for others. You're better off doing a varied full-body routine 3 days a week, altering the exercises every few weeks. That way, you're still regularly challenging your muscles in new ways, but you aren't spending hours upon hours with your weights.

I also prefer full-body workouts over splits because, frankly, it's less easy to screw up your workout schedule. Ideally, you want to work each muscle 2 or 3 days a week. That's easy if you're doing full-body routines. But if you're splitting it up and you miss a day or two of your routine, it's easy to get out of sync and have some muscles go unworked for 6 or 7 days at a stretch.

All about Reps and Sets

Repetitions (or reps for short) refers to the number of times you lift a weight or perform an exercise. Squatting down and up once is considered one repetition. Squatting 10 times would be 10 reps. Sets refers to the number of times you perform those reps. You might do 2 sets of 10 reps, for example. How many reps and sets you do of any given exercise influences how strong and toned your muscle will become.

The Perfectly Fit System sets the target number of repetitions at 10 to 15, beginning with 10 to 12 and working up to 12 to 15. That range helps develop nice gains in strength, muscular endurance (meaning you can do more work before fatiguing), and of course, muscle tone. There's been much research and debate over the ideal number of sets. I suggest two. Studies show that women definitely achieve gains by doing just one set. After that, you can achieve moderate additional gains by adding a second set, and fewer gains by tacking on a third. Considering the additional time it takes for a third set and the law of diminishing returns, do one or two sets and get on with your life.

Sure, there are exceptions. If you were gunning for Amazonian muscle development and brute strength, you would use a heavy weight that you could lift for only 6 to 8 reps and perform multiple (three to five) sets. For more muscular endurance, you would use a lighter weight that you could lift up to 20 times before fatiguing and stick to one to two sets. Endurance lifting won't build much strength or develop muscle, but it can be useful to improve how long your strength lasts in sports like tennis.

There are also countless ways to perform sets, if you're an experimental kinda gal.

Drop sets. Start with your usual weight for an exercise and complete a full set. Then *without* hesitating, pick up the next lowest weight and complete as many reps as you can until you become fatigued. It's a quick, efficient way to challenge your muscles.

between
YOU&ME

Pyramid sets. This is a multiset approach where you start with a low weight at high repetitions for your first set, progressively increase the weight and lower the reps for the next two sets, then come back down the pyramid, lowering weight and increasing reps until you reach the starting point.

Super sets. These are two back-to-back sets of different exercises that work either the same muscle group (upper and lower chest) or opposing muscle groups (chest and back).

Circuits. Do one set of each exercise in your routine without stopping to rest between sets. If necessary, you can take a rest of about 2 minutes, then go through them all again. This is also a good cardio workout.

Running the rack. This is like a super-duper drop set. Start with a heavy weight, fatigue your muscle, drop to the next lowest, fatigue your muscle, and keep on dropping and fatiguing until you're down to the lowest weight available.

These are just fun ways you can vary your routine from time to time. There's no concrete ev-idence that any one system is better than the others. As long as you continue to challenge your muscles with new exercises and moderately heavy weights, you can stick to the standard two-set approach and get great results.

Rest and Recovery: Take Time to Rebuild

Here's a fact that still hasn't sunk in for many elite athletes—you make your advances while you're recovering, not while you're out pushing yourself. Got that? If you want to see improvements in your strength, stamina, and muscle tone, it's important to give your body time to rebuild. The Perfectly Fit workout gives 2 days.

During a lifting session, your muscle fibers actually develop microscopic tears. Although it sounds kind of nasty, this is actually a good thing, because when those fibers heal, they come back stronger. That's the science of strength training. But the key is, you have to let them heal. It takes 48 hours for your muscles to repair, which is why you shouldn't train the same muscles 2 days in a row. This is also why it's important to lift a weight that is heavy enough to challenge your muscles, so you can stimulate this breaking down and re-building process.

Note: Recovery day does not equal lounge-on-the-sofa-and-eat-potato-chips day. It simply means you aren't punishing your freshly trained muscles. You can still go for an easy jog or a bike ride or enjoy some other activity.

The other recovery issue is how much rest you need between sets during your workout. The Perfectly Fit System recommends 20 seconds. By not taking long breaks, you enhance the aerobic component of your workout, and you also don't spend all day with your weights. The only time you would rest longer is if you became involved in serious power lifting, but that's another book.

As Easy as 1-2-3

There are two phases of a repetition—the concentric, or lifting, phase and the eccentric, or lowering, phase. When done properly, both of these phases can help strengthen and tone your muscles.

The most important thing to remember is to lift and lower *slowly*. Go to any weight room and you'll see many people lifting and lowering so rapidly, they look like they're preparing for takeoff. Lifting quickly is a mistake because you use more momentum than muscle to do the work. You also lose the benefits of the eccentric (lowering) phase of the lift. The easiest way to pace yourself properly is to count while you lift. Each rep should take 6 to 7 seconds total. So count 1-2-3 as you lift, pause, then 1-2-3 as you lower. By doing this, you'll be sure to fatigue the maximum number of muscle fibers, and you'll get better results from your efforts. If you're feeling really patient, you can lift even slower, taking 14 seconds per repetition. In a study of 73 men and women, those who completed sets at 14 seconds per lift increased their strength almost 50 percent over those who did each rep at half that speed. Lifting that slowly is tough to do, and I'd never stretch it out that long. But this is a great illustration of how, when it comes to strength training, slower is often better.

Remember also to breathe while you count, exhaling as you push the weight against gravity, and inhaling as you move with gravity. Sounds simple. But it's amazing how many people forget this, hold their breath, and wonder why they feel dizzy.

The Importance of Form

If there has ever been an argument for hiring a personal trainer for at least a session or two, it's learning proper strength-training form. Lifting with poor form is not only less effective than lifting the right way but also, over time, it can cause injuries. Form is particularly important for women because we're generally more flexible than men, which puts us at a higher risk for injury from the get-go. But there's no need to stress about that; proper form is easy to learn. You just need to remember a few simple rules.

Keep your chin up. The first step to good form is keeping your head up and your eyes facing forward. When your head is up and your neck is straight, the rest of your spine is more likely to be in line. Hanging a mirror where you lift helps remind you to do this.

Relax. You should challenge only the muscles you're working while you lift, not your entire body. Keep your jaw, neck, and face relaxed. Hold your shoulders back and relaxed, not shrugged up by your ears. Grasp the weights firmly, but not in a white-knuckle death grip. The less tension you have in your body, the more energy you have to perform your routine.

Focus. Strength-training exercises work better when you focus on the muscle that is doing the work. During a chest press, for instance, concentrate on squeezing the pectoral muscles and using your chest to do most of the work. If you start daydreaming about next month's vacation, it's easy to start simply going through the motions.

Soften up. Your elbows and knees should always remain slightly bent, or soft, and supportive. Don't lock your joints, or even worse, hyperextend them, which is easy for women to do because of our high flexibility.

Remain neutral. Your back works best in its neutral position. That means standing straight, allowing your spine to fall into its normal S curve. Avoid tucking your pelvis forward or arching your back, as that can put too much stress on your vertebrae. Keep your joints neutral as well. Your wrists should be straight, shoulders back and down, and head and neck in line with your spine.

Lift with your legs. You don't use your back to lift heavy boxes, and you shouldn't use it to lift your weights, either. Bend your knees, keep your back neutral, and use your legs to lift.

Watch your knees. Moves that require squatting and knee bending give you killer legs, but they can also be killer on your knees if done improperly. Don't let your knees travel forward out past your toes during squats and lunges. Bend your legs at a 90-degree angle, keeping your knees directly above your ankles.

Keep It Fresh

As you progress in your routine, your body will begin to adapt to it by getting stronger, firmer, and more balanced. Exercises that were once difficult will become easier to do, and you'll feel more confident in your ability. Enjoy this moment. Then move on and change your routine so it is challenging again. Doing the same biceps curls the same way week in and week out will cease to be effective once your body has completely adapted to the exercise. Change your hand position or the angle of the exercise, and suddenly they'll start working again. Maybe more important, you'll be less likely to get bored and quit.

The Perfectly Fit System relies on constant changes in your routine. You'll find a wide variety of exercises for each body part, and you'll find sample ways to put the exercises together. Once you get more comfortable with the system, you'll be able to mix and match on your own. (See chapter 25.)

gearing up for the new muscle movement

This ain't your dad's weight room

When I first started lifting, women in the weight room were a rare species. When you did spy one, she either was with her boyfriend or was a hardcore body builder. Even as recently as 5 years ago, men far outnumbered women, as many women were still intimidated by all the testosterone-laden grunting and weight pounding.

As more women became involved in sports and fitness training, more discovered the body-sculpting wonders of weight training, and a few brave women led the way. As the gym climate changed and word spread, more women followed. Today, it's not uncommon to walk into a gym or club and find more women than men curling dumbbells and pressing weights.

The Women's Movement

For as far as we've come, we still have a long way to go. Not only are there still too few women taking advantage of the body-shaping, fat-burning benefits of resistance

between
YOU&ME

Need more evidence that women and muscles make a sexy marriage? Check out today's supermodels. From swimsuit stunner Rebecca Romijn-Stamos to mainstream model Cindy Crawford, the reigning icons of beauty today all have strong biceps and great abs. Speaking of reigning icons of beauty, it's a little known fact that Marilyn Monroe used dumbbells to maintain her killer curves. Talk about a woman before her time.

training, most women don't understand the wide array of options that are available to them beyond traditional gym equipment.

Barbells, dumbbells, and weight machines are highly effective training tools, without a doubt. But they're not the only, nor always the best, equipment on the block. Women can also take advantage of weighted balls, resistance bands, body bars, and even just their own body weight to work out and get excellent results. And you can use all of this equipment *at home*, which is always a big plus for women who aren't into the gym-rat scene.

Finally, there are new approaches to strength training, like the Perfectly Fit System, that break away and go beyond traditional bodybuilding. Because many women learn strength training from boyfriends and husbands or from male-defined programs, they often get locked into some old-school bodybuilding plans that can get dull, or worse, not even target the areas that women care about most. Plus, many of those traditional pump-you-up plans aren't safe or effective for women's specific joint and muscle needs.

The following chapters will introduce you to the best weight-training tools and techniques available to you. You'll learn what they are, how to use them, and what special benefits they provide, as well as how to work them into a body-shaping, resistance-training program. Then you'll find dozens of exercises to target each and every part of your body. When we put it all together in part 5, you'll find fun and effective ways to get the strength you need and the body you want.

medicine balls

The shaping of the future

L ike tube tops and capri pants, fitness-training techniques come in and out of style. Medicine balls are the latest training tools to make a comeback, but unlike the chunky leather medicine balls from 30 years ago, today's medicine balls come in a large variety of textures, weights, and sizes. They're symmetrical and fun to use, and they can tone and shape in ways that traditional weight equipment can't.

Popularly used for sports training and in Olympic training centers, medicine balls are showing up increasingly in mainstream fitness magazines, health clubs, and classes. When medicine balls aren't available, you can often substitute a dumbbell, but they don't work quite as well. If the exercise involves any kind of tossing or throwing motion, you're better off sticking with a medicine ball, or even a basketball or volleyball.

Unique Benefits

Medicine balls have many unique benefits, but the one that most women (and men) like best is the ab toning. Tossing a ball in the air between crunches is a fast way to tighten your midriff. And most medicine ball exercises require that you contract your abs for stability and balance, which gives your abs a bonus workout throughout your routine.

Awesome abs aside, maybe the greatest thing about medicine balls is that they train your body for real-life activity, giving you what is known as functional fitness. This is especially important because it's during simple daily chores like lifting awk-

between
YOU&ME

Medicine balls are my favorite way to work out. There's something about the shape and feel that is both feminine and strong at the same time. Curl your hands around one, and you feel like the Muscle Goddess holding the world in your hands. Wield your power, girl!

ward-shaped bags or carrying children that we tend to get hurt. We all know that we should lift with our legs and not with our backs, for instance, but have you ever tried to get a baby out of a crib without using your lower back? Medicine balls allow for a wide range of motion and let you move your hands, arms, back, and legs in ways that closely mimic these everyday tasks. They also build and strengthen your supporting muscles, joints, and ligaments to respond quickly to the demands of an active life.

If you play any kind of sports or physical activities, medicine ball training will help you play better. Medicine ball exercises strengthen your core, or the center of your body, including your abs, back, and hips, so you have more power and balance for running, jumping, throwing, and striking with a bat or a racket. Plus, you can simulate almost any sports move—from a golf swing to a softball toss—to strengthen the exact muscles you use in the exact way you use them.

Completely unscientifically, tossing around these bright, colorful balls is just fun. Once some people try them, they don't want to go back to

dumbbells and weight machines. I think they're a good complement for each other.

Choosing the Right Ball for You

It used to be that there wasn't much choice when it came to medicine balls. You got big, heavy, and leather. No more. Today's medicine balls range from tennis-ball size to bigger than a basketball. They come as light as 1 pound and as heavy as 30 pounds. And while you can still buy soft leather balls, you can also buy balls that bounce, balls with handles, plastic balls, and rubber balls.

What's the best ball for your workout? For most exercises, 4 to 6 pounds is plenty. If you're already active in strength training, you may go as high as 10 pounds. But even strong women can get a workout from a fairly light ball because the moves tend to involve multiple muscle groups.

As for size, the ball should fit comfortably between both hands, either a volleyball or softball size. The texture is a matter of personal choice. Just be sure that the surface is "grippy" enough that the ball doesn't easily slip from your hands.

You can get a basic leather medicine ball from Champion (check your local sporting goods chain stores) for under $20. Or you can order them from companies such as Perform Better (800-556-7464), Power Systems (800-321-6975), or JumpUSA (800-586-7872).

Special Tips

Medicine ball training is more dynamic than traditional weight training, as you bend, twist, turn, and

PERFECTLY FIT IDEAS

There are medicine ball exercises throughout this book, but once you get the hang of them, it's fun to make up your own. Try these.

Tosses. You can strengthen your tendons and ligaments by tossing the ball up in the air and catching it. Add tosses into squats by tossing the ball when you're in the standing position and catching it as you go into your squat. Add a toss between ab crunches to make your stomach muscles work double duty as you contract to push the ball away and then again to absorb the impact.

Passes. Grab a partner and practice some passing drills. Hold the ball at chest height and push your arms forward, passing the ball from your chest to work your arms, shoulders, and chest muscles. Start from a squat with the ball in front of your chest and spring up and toss the ball to work your legs and butt. Hold the ball down by your right hip, twist your torso, and throw the ball in a shoveling motion to work your abdominals and obliques. Or swing the ball between your legs and throw the ball forward as you come up to work your back and legs.

Swings and twists. Swinging and twisting exercises are ideal for golf, softball, or racquet sports players because they strengthen the muscles throughout your torso, including your obliques and lower back. Hold the ball in front of you and twist from side to side to strengthen bat-swinging muscles. Swing it over alternate shoulders to mimic a golf swing.

Balancing tricks. Improve your strength and balance by doing pushups with your hands or feet on a ball. Try balancing on one foot on a ball for 30 seconds. If necessary, stand by a wall for support in case you lose balance. Test your limits. Then push them.

---

toss. It's easy to overdo it. So learning to use proper form and technique is important for the best results. The following tips can help.

Start slowly. Because medicine ball workouts involve so much bending and twisting, it's important to begin with a light weight and start slowly to build your delicate lower-back muscles and supporting tendons and ligaments. Stick to one set of 10 to 12 repetitions for the first few weeks, and progress to two sets of 12 to 15 reps when the exercises have become less challenging.

Relax and give. Tossing and catching the medicine ball, either by yourself or with a partner, is a key part of medicine ball training. But remember, these aren't airy rubber balls; they have some weight to them. When throwing a medicine ball, bend your knees and put your whole body behind it. When catching one, relax your hands and "give" with your elbows, bringing the ball to your body, to absorb the impact. Start with gentle lobs, to get the feeling of catching a weighted ball before you toss higher or with more force.

Remember to rest. Medicine ball workouts really stimulate the central nervous system, especially once you start tossing and catching. You'll actually feel a bit of a buzz when you're done. This is great for keeping your coordination and reflexes sharp, but a little goes a long way. Take 48 hours off between workouts to give your body time to recover fully.

bands and tubing

Tone and go

Confession: I always thought resistance bands were for wimps. Like so many strength-training snobs, I couldn't take them seriously. Then I started teaching a sculpt-and-tone class where the only tools available were balls, bands, and light dumbbells. A day of achy muscles later, I saw that my attitude was out of line. Bands *can* give even "serious" women a serious workout.

Rubber resistance bands as well as rubber tubing have been around for decades. Originally just big gray strips of latex used by physical therapists to help people regain strength after injury, today's resistance strips and tubes come in a wide variety of colorful options. There are minibands, long bands, short bands, tubes with handles, tubes with poles—all available from the easiest to the most difficult resistance. All can give you a great workout.

Unique Benefits

Portability is the greatest benefit of resistance bands. No other fitness equipment stashes away so easily in a suitcase or a handbag to give you an on-the-go gym. When I meet with women who travel for a living, I always give them an exercise band. They can do a whole-body strength-training workout when they're on the road, even if there's not a dumbbell within 50 miles of their hotels.

Bands and tubes are also remarkably versatile. Unlike free weights, where you need a variety of weights to complete a workout, you can adjust the resistance on a band or tube by simply choking up on it to make it more difficult or lengthening your grip placement to make it easier.

You'll also find that even though bands don't work your muscles quite as hard as free weights do, they give your muscles less rest, making them work longer. That's because unlike weights that rely on gravity for resistance, bands and tubes provide their own constant resistance as long as you're holding them taut. This allows you to challenge your muscles in a wider range of motion.

So why don't we use bands for everything? The constant tension of bands makes some moves—especially overhead presses and exercises where the weight is high on the body—awkward to perform. The bands tend to pull your arms out to the sides more than gravity does when you're trying to push out or up in a straight line. And it can be difficult to get enough resistance from them for certain large-muscle exercises like leg presses. For lower-body toning exercises like leg lifts, however, they can actually be superior to weights.

Choosing the Right Resistance for You

The selection of resistance bands and tubes can be downright dizzying. Don't let yourself be oversold, however. You really only need one or two simple strips of latex. The rest are frills. Here's a

rundown on the products available and what they're good for.

Straight bands. These are simple strips of latex that come in a variety of resistance from light to "special heavy." It's best to go with a medium-resistance band that you can choke up to make harder or let out to make easier. Choose a long band (6 feet or longer) to allow for the greatest variety of exercises. Or buy two so you can tie them together. They're especially good for back and leg exercises. Two well-known brands are Dyna-Band and Thera-Band.

Looped bands. Like large rubber bands, looped bands are a thicker, narrower cut of rubber than the very light and wide straight bands. Looped around your ankles, these bands give a screaming glute and leg workout. They're available in a range of sizes and resistance from shorter bands (about 9 inches long) to longer bands (20 to 56 inches long) with light to heavy resistance. Your best bet is to buy a shorter band with medium resistance.

Tubing. The most sophisticated of the resistance rubber products, tubing comes in a variety of resistance from light to super heavy (again, medium is usually a good bet if you're buying just one). Unlike bands, tubing is available with attachments like handles, plastic poles (to use as barbells), ankle straps, and door anchors. These accessories make it easier to handle the tubing as you would a free weight, but it also makes it a little more work to adjust the resistance and to switch from exercise to exercise, because you have to change attachments. Obviously, tubing also costs a little more because of the accessories, but it's still fairly cheap.

Bungee cords. Strong, cloth-covered stretchy bungee cord comes with a clip on one end and a hand strap on the other. It's not very practical for most exercises, and the most expensive of the bunch.

My recommendation is to buy one long straight band and one medium-resistance looped band, and for about $10 you'll have a quick home gym that's simple to use. You can buy the bands at almost any sporting goods store, or you can order them from companies such as Perform Better (800-556-7464) and Power Systems (800-321-6975).

Special Tips

To get the most out of resistance band training, proper form is essential—as is care for your equipment. The following tips can help.

Pull steadily. In freeweight lifting, the resistance is toughest at midlift and easier in both the starting and final positions (a squat is easiest when you're squatting and standing, but toughest in the transition). But a band's resistance becomes progressively more difficult from beginning to end and doesn't ease up in the final position. This can make you feel a little wobbly the first few times. Concentrate on moving slowly and steadily against the resistance, performing your reps in a smooth, continuous motion.

Perform a prelift inspection. Give your bands a quick once-over for rips and tears before you start your exercise routine. Though it's not common, sometimes they snap. And you know that's gotta hurt.

Step firmly. Some exercises require that you hold your exercise band down with your feet while lifting the other end. If you're stepping with only one foot, be sure to step very firmly with your heel, or even better, tie the band securely around your foot. Again, no one wants to get snapped with a flying 6-foot band!

Baby your bands. Once a month, put your bands or tubes in a plastic bag, sprinkle in some baby powder, and shake them up to coat them. This will help prolong the life of the rubber.

Exercise on the Go

My job sometimes requires that I travel for days on end. Here's a great band routine that I use in my hotel room to keep from getting grumpy and sluggish because I can't work out. If you're new to strength training, you can do fewer repetitions and sets of all of the exercises, starting with one set in the 10 to 12 range.

Exercise	Reps	Sets
Lat pulldown (p. 138)	12 to 15	2
Seated row (p. 74)	12 to 15	2
Single-arm crossover (p. 148)	10 to 12	2
Rubber band sidestep (p. 109)	10 to 12	2
Monster walk (p. 111)	10 to 12	2
Seated inner-leg lift (p. 120) (no band)	10 to 12	2
2-second floor crunch (no band) (p. 126)	15 to 20	2

body-weight resistance

No equipment required

t's the oldest form of strength training. Before there were barbells, Nautilus, and Bowflex, there were arms, legs, and the torso that's attached. And that was (and still is) enough to tone your body into top form. And if you play sports or are at all physically active, body weight training is a great way to make sure you can—quite literally—pull your own weight.

More good news: Body weight exercises like pushups, dips, and pullups are surging in popularity, especially among women, after a few years of being scorned as too boring, difficult, or military-like. More women are discovering that a few well-designed routines can be a fun, effective, and superconvenient way to work out. The trick is knowing how to do them. I've included a variety of body weight exercises in parts 2 and 3, along with full instructions. With a little more understanding of how they work, you can develop a routine (or adapt an existing one) that's suited just for you.

Unique Benefits

Hands down, the biggest benefit of body weight exercises is convenience. You do not have to go to a gym to do them, and you don't need any equipment. That means no matter what kind of curveball life throws your way, from extended business trips to family vacations, you can keep your strength-training routine—and your muscle tone—without missing a beat.

What's more, pushing and pulling your own body weight can really boost your confidence. Women totally *glow* after polishing off a set of pushups or completing a full pullup for the first time, and I don't just mean from exertion. It's an accomplishment that gives you the sense that you are strong enough to kick some butt. And that kind of self-assurance shines through in everything you do.

On the most practical level, there is no better way to ensure that you will be able to live strongly and independently, getting up from chairs and out of bed with ease well into your old age, than by regularly performing body weight exercises like squats, curl ups, and dips. These exercises use the muscles you need for daily living and mimic your everyday moves. The same, of course, applies to playing sports. Nothing prepares you better for hefting your own weight around than hefting your own weight around. It's that simple.

Cosmetically speaking, body weight exercises are ideal for shaping and toning. Leg lifts, stomach crunches, lunges, and squats put your major muscle groups to the test, which not only firms and tones your muscles but also burns a fair number of calories (almost 400 calories per hour for a 140-pound woman), so you'll shed more unwanted fat, too.

Choosing Your Space

Forget about high-tech equipment and special gear. All you need for body weight exercises are a

roomy area and a few bare-bones items. Speaking of bare, you may be tempted to work out in your bare feet, but don't. Workout shoes, like those for walking, running, or cross-training, provide cushioning and structure for better balance and support. Plus, lacing up your shoes sends a signal to your brain that you're ready to exercise, and you're more likely to take your workout seriously.

Besides shoes, here are a few things to include when setting up your space.

A carpet or mat. Since many body weight exercises are done on the floor, you'll want some padding to soften the pressure on your hips, knees, and back. Any room with a well-padded carpet will do the trick. In the case of hardwood floors, you'll want to buy an exercise mat (they're under $20 and available at any discount or fitness store) or at least place a folded towel under high-contact areas such as your knees during pushups.

A stable chair. A sturdy chair is a home gym on its own. It provides support for triceps dips, leg extensions, squats, hip hikes, and even ab crunches. Try to find one without arms and with an unpadded seat. Your basic wooden chair works best.

A sturdy table. While not as important as a chair, a solid table or desk can give a boost to your body weight workouts. You can lean against it for modified pushups. You can hang beneath it for modified pullups. And it can provide support for leg lifts, side kicks, and other standing exercises.

Special Tips

The trickiest part of body weight workouts is adapting the exercises and routine to suit your personal strength and fitness needs. With traditional weight lifting, it's easy. You just grab the right weight for you and do your sets. When that weight becomes too easy, you lift a heavier one. But how do you adjust your workout when some exercises become so easy you can do 50 while others remain too tough to do even one? The answer is to do them smarter. Here's how.

Slow it down. So you can do 15 abdominal crunches without blinking. Try slowing down each rep, taking 4 seconds to raise and 4 seconds to lower, and see how much harder 15 reps become. By slowing down the pace of your exercises, you lose momentum and force your muscles to work even harder.

Adjust your levers. Exercises like pushups and dips often frustrate women (who naturally have less upper-body strength than men) because they think they're too hard. But these exercises are easily adapted to any level of strength. The key is adjusting how much of your body you are lifting. Take a pushup as an example. When you're up on your toes, your chest and arms are pressing every ounce. Bend your legs and push up from your knees, and suddenly the exercise is more manageable.

Add mini-reps. Make an exercise harder without adding sets or reps simply by holding the move midway and "pulsing," or doing several mini-reps. During a squat, for example, try stopping halfway between your standing and squatting point and moving up and down ever so slightly for 5 to 10 seconds.

Work the angles. To maximize the number of muscle fibers you challenge—and to get better toning—change the angle of your exercises to work the same muscles in a new way. Do leg lifts lying down for a few weeks. Then do them standing up. Place your hands closer together or farther away during pushups. These tiny tricks make big differences in the way you use your muscles.

Think smaller sets. We're so used to shooting for 10 to 15 repetitions, it's hard to imagine that just 4 or 5 reps could do any good. But in the case of body weight exercises, they can. If you can just eke out five pushups, then that's your set. Try to do the same in the second set. Eventually, you'll do six pushups, and then seven, and then . . . you get the picture.

Exercise on the Go

There's something sexy and satisfying about banging out some pushups and pullups in the hotel while you're on vacation. This on-the-go routine is my favorite. If you're new to strength training, you can do fewer repetitions and sets of all of the exercises, starting with one set in the 10 to 12 rep range.

Exercise	Reps	Sets
Squat and side lift (p. 86)	10 to 15	2
Pushup (p. 70)	10 to 12	2
Pullup (p. 79)	10 to 12	2
Chair dip (p. 80)	10 to 12	2
Chair curl (p. 127)	15 to 20	2
Dog walk (p. 104)	12 to 15	2
Side-lying side kick (p. 105)	12 to 15	2
Flamingo hip twist (p. 110)	10 to 12	2
Seated straight-leg lift (p. 114)	12 to 15	2
Superwoman (p. 141)	10 to 12	2

free weights

The best of the basics

For supersexy muscle tone and a fully functional body, nothing beats free weights. *Free weights*—the common term for dumbbells, barbells, and ankle weights—work your muscles like you do in real life, lifting against and resisting the force of gravity. Unlike machines, free weights also force you to stabilize your body as you lift and lower, so you develop better balance and stronger supporting muscles, joints, and ligaments. Plus, they can work each muscle from almost every conceivable angle, so you get total-muscle toning.

Because of their superior convenience and versatility, I prefer dumbbells to barbells. Here are just a few of the special benefits these free weights provide, advice on how to pick the right weights for you, and tips for using them correctly.

Unique Benefits

One of the best things about dumbbells and ankle weights is that each limb has to pull its own weight during your routine. Since you can't favor your stronger side, like you can using machines, you end up with a more balanced body. Many women I train are surprised at how much weaker their left sides are (when they're right-handed) compared to their right. Dumbbells and ankle weights help even out those muscular imbalances.

They also mimic real life. Just as you lift boxes, put away groceries, and push and pull heavy doors, free weight exercises demand that you curl, reach, pull, and

between
YOU&ME

press to strengthen those much-used muscles. Even better: Unlike machines that lock you in a fixed position, free weights require that you stabilize yourself as you perform the exercises. You get the added benefit of stronger core muscles like abs and back as well as stronger stabilizing muscles and connective tissues.

Want to shape your shoulders? Build up your biceps? Tone your inner thighs? It doesn't get any easier than with dumbbells. Free weights allow you to target the exact muscle that you want to tone. And though it's a controversial point, I find that they give better muscle development than pricey machines and exercise equipment. Many times I've worked with women and men who have been "doing Nautilus" for months, even years, but haven't seen much change in their bodies. After a few weeks with dumbbells, we get definition.

Finally, dumbbells offer more bang for your buck than almost any other fitness equipment money can buy. For less than $100, you can buy all the weights you'll ever need, and there are literally hundreds of dumbbell and ankle weight exercises you can do—many of which you'll find right here.

Choosing the Right Weights for You

As resistance training's popularity climbs steadily the selection of free weights on the fitness store shelves continues to expand. Where your choices were once limited to gray metal or gray metal, today's dumbbells come in a wide array of shapes, sizes, and materials.

What's the best weight for you? If you're looking for cheap, durable weights, standard steel

PERFECTLY FIT IDEAS

You'll find dozens of free weight exercises throughout the book. But once you get a feel for them, you can start making personal adaptations to your routines. Here are some ideas to try.

Flip your grip. Once you're very comfortable with the standard exercises, you can experiment with different hand positions and see how they work your muscles in a whole new way. Try performing a biceps curl with your palm facing down rather than up, and you'll feel the difference immediately.

Go to the bars. If you own or have access to a barbell or weighted body bar, go ahead and substitute it for your dumbbells for exercises like chest presses, arm curls, and squats. It'll work your muscles in a new way and provide a fresh change.

is still your best bet. You can expect to pay 40 to 50 cents a pound, depending on the quality of the metal and construction, and they should last forever. Cold metal not your preference? Pick up a pair of vinyl-coated dumbbells. They're available in bright colors and are pleasant to the touch, but usually are not available in weights heavier than 10 pounds. The most recent additions to the dumbbell family are soft, flexible weights called Lei Weights. These weights look like flat, canvas dumbbells, but don't be fooled. They flop around too much to use for most dumbbell exercises. What they are good for is draping across different body parts to add resistance during exercises like pushups, dips, and leg raises.

How many weights do you need? While you don't need a full rack, I do recommend buying more than one set. Ideally, you need three sets: One set of very light weights for small muscles such as shoulders (you probably won't need a weight that is less than 3 pounds, however), one set of medium for arm curls and chest presses, and one set of heavier weights for squats and lunges. Remember, the weight should be heavy enough so the last 3 or 4 repetitions are tough and you can't lift past 15.

Whatever weights you choose, I recommend picking up a set of PlateMates to go with them. These are small magnetic weights you stick on the end of a dumbbell to increase its weight in 1- to 3-pound increments. They're perfect for increasing the weight for small-muscle exercises, where a 5-pound increment may be too much.

For your lower body, strap-on ankle weights are best. Choose a pair that is adjustable up to 10

BARBELLS AND BODY BARS

Barbells and weighted body bars are also included in the "free weight" category. Barbells are simply metal bars that you can slip weighted plates onto for exercises like presses, rows, and squats. Body bars are a less sophisticated alternative, as the bar itself is designed to provide all the weight you need. They're usually vinyl-coated and used for less intense exercises than barbells are. Both are great for shaping and toning muscles, but because they aren't as convenient or versatile as dumbbells, I don't suggest bars as part of the Perfectly Fit System—though you can substitute them for curls and presses if you have one. If you're interested in buying a barbell for home use, I recommend the Soft Stick. It's a foam-covered barbell that allows you to slip soft weights on the end, taking the bar from 12 pounds to 24 pounds. Look for it in sporting goods stores.

pounds. (Adjustable weights have slotted pockets for putting in or taking out 1-pound weighted bars.)

Special Tips

Free weights work best when used with correct form. Sloppy technique will give you fewer benefits and can also lead to muscle or joint injuries. Fortunately, proper form is easy to learn. Just follow the instructions given with each exercise, and apply the following tips.

Master the form first. Always use a very light weight the first time you try an exercise. You want to concentrate on getting the form down first. Once you're comfortable with the technique, you can add the appropriate weight to challenge your muscles.

Avoid the dead zones. Free weights supply what is known as dynamic constant resistance. This is just a fancy way of saying that the amount of force on your muscle changes through the exercise because of the changing relationship with gravity. During a biceps curl, for example, there's little to no resistance in the starting position or at the very top of the lift. But there's plenty in between. To get the most out of your free weight workout, avoid those "dead zones" where there's no load on your muscles, and keep the weight in a range of constant tension.

Use muscle, not momentum. Lift too quickly and you'll gain so much momentum that your muscles will miss their workout. Count 1-2-3 as you lift and 1-2-3 as you lower, and you'll use more muscle power and less momentum. You'll feel—and see—the difference.

combination moves

Twice the toning in half the time

'll be the first to admit it: Traditional bodybuilding can get dull. You lift the weight. You lower the weight. You repeat. That's why so many women fall away from their programs after the first few months. It's not that they aren't seeing results; it's that they're bored. I was too, until I discovered a new way of lifting—a way that's fun, mentally challenging, and makes more sense for the way our bodies move. This new technique is called combination lifting. It absorbs all of the old single-muscle moves and morphs them into multimove exercises that challenge and tone twice the muscles in half the time.

Easy combination moves like squat raises, lunge kicks, and curl and presses add a refreshing challenge to beginner programs, while more advanced moves help experienced lifters turbo their toning to the next level. Once you get the hang of how to do them and how they work, you might even find yourself creating some combination moves of your own.

Unique Benefits

One of the biggest draws of combination moves for time-pressed women is their sheer efficiency. Instead of doing two individual sets of triceps kickbacks for each arm, then two sets of hip extensions for each leg, you bring them together, toning

You'll find dozens of combination moves throughout this book, along with programs for putting them together. But once you get a feel for them, you can start creating your own routines and adjusting existing routines to your liking. Here are some ideas to try.

String them together. Strapped for time? String together 10 to 15 combination moves for a light, body-sculpting aerobic workout. Simply move through the series of exercises, without stopping, two or three times—I guarantee you'll sweat up a storm.

Move to music. Combination moves go well with music; it almost feels as though you're dancing as you lunge, press, squat, and curl. Just make sure the music isn't too fast. African or Cuban dance music provides a good steady beat, as do most dance club tracks. But steer clear of traditional "aerobics" music—it's too high speed, and it's usually annoying.

Mix your own moves. Play tennis, golf, or some other sport? String together some moves that mimic the actions of your activity. Combine moves that work your glutes, deltoids, hamstrings, and obliques, for instance, and you'll strengthen those muscles and connective tissues you use while placing the ball and taking a swing in golf. Let your creativity be your guide.

both the upper body and the lower body in one fluid move. As one client put it, "Now it'll take me *no* time to finish my workout!"

Because combination moves often work mus-cles in your upper and lower body simultaneously, they also strengthen your core abdominal and back muscles because you have to contract those muscles throughout the exercise to maintain balance and form. The result is finely toned abs and a strong, straight back.

Too often I hear women complain that they are uncoordinated—undoubtedly a label that was tattooed on their psyches back in junior high gym class. Combination moves improve coordination and boost confidence, as women find that with a little practice and some added muscle power, they really can move with grace and strength.

Like so many exercises in the Perfectly Fit System, combination moves mimic real life. Think of how your body moves while stashing your carry-on luggage on a plane. You squat to pick up the carry-on, you curl it to your shoulders, then you press it into the overhead. That's a classic real-life combination move, and it's the kind of challenge these exercises prepare your body to perform.

All those serious benefits aside, the thing I like best about combination exercises is that they feel like play. I teach a class that is almost entirely combination moves put to music. The women have so much fun lungeing, kicking, and curling that they're still smiling as they head to the showers, and still ragging on me for torturing them.

Special Tips

Combination moves are more involved and dynamic than most traditional weight-training exercises. Because they challenge your muscles (and coordination) in new ways, you'll need some prac-

between
YOU&ME

tice before you get the hang of them. The following tips can help.

Focus on the working muscles. Each exercise description tells you what muscles are being challenged by the move. To get the most out of each exercise, focus on contracting and using those specific muscles during the move. By concentrating on the muscles that are supposed to do the work, you're less likely to slip into sloppy form

or rely on other, maybe stronger, muscles to complete the exercise.

Don't forgo form. Because they command more muscles with every move, combination exercises can be more fatiguing than traditional weight-training moves. Ultimately, you want to work up to 12 to 15 repetitions of many of these exercises, but you probably won't start there. And you shouldn't let your good form lapse just to eke out the final 4 repetitions. Do as many reps as you can with proper technique, and as soon as you feel your form starting to fall apart—your head drops down, your back arches, your shoulders hunch—stop. Rest for 1 minute and try another set.

Isolate the trouble spots. Combination moves are fun, fast, and effective for total-body toning. But you'll notice that most of the programs in the Perfectly Fit System also incorporate some isolation exercises because the one thing combination moves don't do is allow you to focus all your attention on one particular trouble spot. (And we all have one!) The best routine is a smart combination of both.

PART 2

PERFECTLY
FIT

the
moves

perfectly fit moves for a terrific body

Fast, fun exercises to shape up every inch

Contrary to how many of us look at and treat our bodies, we are more than sums of our separate parts. You are not just thighs, boobs, abs, and arms. You are a chain of beautiful muscles that run, literally, from the top of your head to the bottom of your feet. To get a balanced, toned, Perfectly Fit body, you have to engage your entire body regularly, using all those beautiful muscles, not just picking a few to work over and over and over again.

This is a hard lesson to learn for most of us. I too once thought I could attain the ultimate tush if I just did 5,332 leg lifts a day. Like so many women, I would single-mindedly focus on the parts I wanted to "fix," ignoring those that were holding their own. The result was a lot of work for very little reward. Then I discovered integrative, multimuscle moves like those used by many professional athletes and their trainers. The idea of working out faster and more efficiently was appealing, so I tried. it. Unbelievably, areas around my hips and love handles, for which I had long since abandoned hope, started shaping up. I began including these exercises in all my programs for clients. Three weeks later, a man who had been striving for a six-pack for 5 years was literally gushing about how firm his stomach was becoming. When he included the rest of his body in the equation, his abs finally got flat.

Three years later, I've compiled dozens and dozens of these fast, efficient, total-body toners. And I've put them together in a Perfectly Fit System.

Active, Balanced Bodies

You'll find more than 90 exercises in this section. The first 40 of them, found in chapter 12, are combination moves that challenge two, three, or sometimes four or more muscle groups per repetition. These are athletic whole-body moves, but you don't have to be an athlete to do them. You'll just look like one when you're done. The rest of this section comprises isolation exercises, which concentrate on one individual muscle group at a time, broken down into specific "goal" chapters such as chapter 13, Perfectly Fit Goal: Shapely, Strong Arms.

What? After my big soliloquy on training as a whole being I go and chop you up into body parts anyway? Not exactly. Even though total-body moves are indeed the heart and soul of Perfectly Fit toning, there *is* a time and place for a few isolation exercises. For one, when you are just starting out, it's common to have some muscle imbalances. Your biceps are probably pretty strong from lifting shopping bags and backpacks, for instance, but your triceps may be totally underused. These

between YOU&ME

I'll be the first to admit it: Some of these exercises are tough to master. Because they challenge your balance and coordination as well as many small supporting muscles that are often neglected, these moves are challenging in a way no biceps curl ever could be. It may be tempting to say, "Forget it," and stick to the easy stuff. Don't. The rewards of pushing through the tough moves are huge. While I wasn't specifically looking to lose weight, since starting these exercise programs myself, I've lost almost 15 pounds and dropped 5 percent body fat. I'm racing faster and feel stronger and lighter than ever. The hard stuff always pays off.

kinds of imbalances can make it tough to perform high-level multimuscle moves. A solid beginning program will include a well-rounded selection of isolation exercises that focus on individual muscles, combined with just one or two simple compound moves. That way, all of the muscles get a basic foundation of strength before they perform together. And, of course, there are people who are generally fit, but have one stubborn area. In those cases, we add specific isolation exercises to a total-body routine to home in on that trouble zone.

Part 3 is designed with all that in mind and provides the right mix of combination and isolation moves for your specific fitness needs. Then you can go ahead and start combining exercises on your own!

Keep It Fresh

You might wonder why I've chosen to put 80, instead of, oh, say 25, exercises in this book. First off, it's important to incorporate a fair amount of variety into your routine on a regular basis to completely develop muscle strength and tone.

It works like this. Your muscles are made up of thousands of fibers. Each exercise recruits a certain number of muscle fibers to complete the effort. Many, but not all, of the fibers are targeted with any given move. To tone and strengthen all of the fibers in a given muscle, therefore, you have to work the muscle in different ways and from different angles to recruit as many fibers as possible.

An example: You do lunges to tone and strengthen your quadriceps. It's a great exercise, but if all you ever did were lunges, you would be targeting only the fibers needed to complete a lunge, and some of your quad muscles would go unchallenged. By changing your routine regularly to incorporate fresh quad exercises, like side to sides, you'll recruit and tone more of your muscle fibers.

I also want this book to last you a long, long time. Maybe your whole life. And as your fitness improves, your exercise goals and needs will change. You'll need new and different exercises to keep your muscles challenged and your mind from getting bored. I recommend shaking things up every 4 weeks for optimum results and enjoyment.

So there's the philosophy behind how it all works. Now it's time to apply it for yourself. Start by taking a few minutes to look through the exercises. Some of them will seem familiar. Many will be completely new to you. Then, flip to part 3 and use the programs that have been prepared for you. Most important: Just get moving and have fun!

total-body toning

40 moves for a perfectly fit body

Some of the most beautiful bodies I've ever seen have been at triathlons. These multisport athletes seem to have it all—strong curvy shoulders, sexy backs, toned abs, and lean legs. They look so stunning because they use every single muscle in their bodies as they stroke through the water, pedal across hilly terrain, and run to the finish. The result is strong, balanced, knockout bodies.

The following 40 exercises are designed to work multiple muscle groups with each exercise. This is the core of the Perfectly Fit System for total-body toning. By working more of your major muscles with every move, you get two big benefits.

One, you save tons of time because each exercise delivers more bang for your buck. Two, you develop more "functional" muscular fitness. Functional fitness is one of the best new trends in the strength-training industry. Rather than concentrating on isolating just one or two muscles per exercise, as in an arm curl for your biceps or a leg extension for your quadriceps, you work multiple muscles together, the way you do in real life. Think about it. You don't pick up a gallon of orange juice and curl it 15 times. You squat down, pick it up off the shelf, and lift it into your cart. That's functional strength. And you need to work on it to get it.

As a bonus, these exercises develop strong core muscles because you need to keep those muscles activated to maintain proper form throughout the moves. In plain language, that means that these exercises will help give you a strong, toned back and great abs and obliques as well. You'll find many exercises here that you've probably never seen before. You'll also find some classic standbys as some of these exercises are too good not to include in your routine.

Getting started. Because they work multiple muscles, these exercises can be pretty fatiguing. If you're new to strength training, the idea is to work these exercises into a full-body routine. If you're an imaginative lifter who's developing your own programs, simply pick and choose the ones you like and work them into your routine. Avoid doing the same exercise 2 days in a row so that your muscles can recover. And start slowly. Do just one set

between YOU&ME

You can do your strength-training routine any time of day that works for you. But I love doing these exercises first thing in the morning (after a brief warmup). Because they stretch and strengthen every muscle in your body, they're a perfect way to get primed to take on the day.

of 10 to 12 repetitions to begin, and work up to two sets of 12 to 15 reps. Rest for 20 seconds between sets. See "Exercise Ratings" on page 48 to determine which level of exercise is best for you.

MUSCLE SPEAK

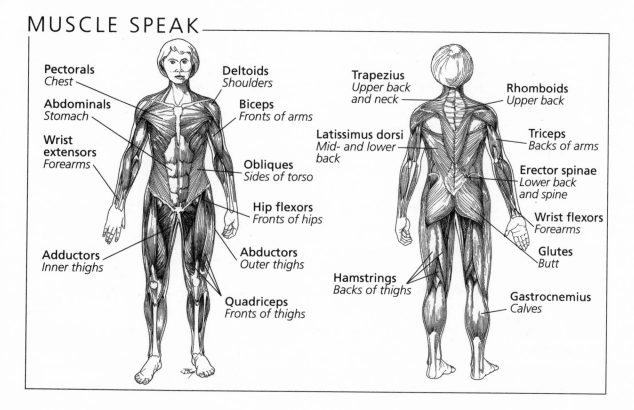

Pectorals
Chest

Abdominals
Stomach

Wrist extensors
Forearms

Adductors
Inner thighs

Deltoids
Shoulders

Biceps
Fronts of arms

Obliques
Sides of torso

Hip flexors
Fronts of hips

Abductors
Outer thighs

Quadriceps
Fronts of thighs

Trapezius
Upper back and neck

Latissimus dorsi
Mid- and lower back

Hamstrings
Backs of thighs

Rhomboids
Upper back

Triceps
Backs of arms

Erector spinae
Lower back and spine

Wrist flexors
Forearms

Glutes
Butt

Gastrocnemius
Calves

MUSCLE REMINDERS

❏ Warm up for 5 to 10 minutes before lifting.
❏ Pick a weight that you can lift for no more than 10 to 15 reps before resting.
❏ The final 2 to 3 reps should be difficult.
❏ Always lift in a slow, controlled manner, counting 3 seconds as you lift, pausing for 1 second, and counting 3 seconds as you lower.
❏ Begin with one set. Work up to two.
❏ When alternating arms or legs throughout an exercise, aim for 20 to 30 reps—10 to 15 reps to a side.

❏ Exhale as you lift and exert. Inhale as you return to the starting position.
❏ An aerobic step is a good investment, since you can use it as a weight bench for lying-down exercises as well as stepping exercises for the lower body. But if you don't have an aerobic step or weight bench, you often can use a firm bed or the floor for the upper-body moves and regular stairs for the lower-body exercises.

What to expect. Expect to feel awkward. Some of these exercises will seem familiar, but many will not. You'll feel a little shaky the first few times, but once your brain develops the new neuromuscular (mind-muscle) connections it needs, you'll feel stronger and more stable. They take a little more coordination than the more traditional exercises, but they work, and if you build up to them, you can definitely do them.

Safety first. Many of these exercises are designed for women who already have some basic strength. If you're just starting out, are out of shape, or have some muscles that are much weaker than others, start with the basic moves. They demand less muscle, torso, and joint stability to be performed safely and correctly. Beginners should include more isolation exercises in their workouts to get muscles up to speed before doing a total combination-move workout.

Results. Perform a full-body routine 3 or 4 days a week, and you'll feel stronger in 2 to 3 weeks. After 4 to 6 weeks, you'll start seeing results.

EXERCISE RATINGS

❏ BASIC: These exercises are good for beginners and seasoned lifters alike. Since they don't require high amounts of coordination, they're ideal for people just starting out. Experienced lifters may find themselves using a little more weight to make these exercises more challenging.

❏ INTERMEDIATE: These exercises challenge balance, coordination, and small supporting muscles. They're best for people who are already fairly active (walking, exercise classes, basic strength training). Beginners can work up to the intermediate exercises after several weeks of a basic training routine.

❏ ADVANCED: These exercises require a fair amount of strength, balance, and coordination to be performed properly. They are best for experienced strength trainers who want a challenge.

Full Body

The following exercises are considered full-body moves because you must use both upper and lower major muscle groups to perform them correctly.

wood chop

Muscles worked: Erector spinae, hamstrings, glutes, and deltoids
Perfectly Fit bonus: Less soreness and fatigue from sitting at a desk all day
Rating: BASIC
Equipment: A medicine ball or dumbbell

Stand with your feet wider than shoulder-width apart, keeping your knees slightly bent. Hold a medicine ball or dumbbell in both hands over your head (1).

Bend at the waist, keeping your back flat, and swing the ball down between your shins as though you're hiking a football (2). Your knees will bend naturally as you do this. Pause, then swing the ball back over your head while simultaneously standing back upright.

Lift Tips

○ Start with a very light weight and a high number of repetitions, such as 1 to 3 pounds and 12 to 15 reps, since this exercise can be demanding on the lower-back muscles, which tend to be weak from underuse.

○ When using a dumbbell instead of a medicine ball, hold the weight with both hands around the bar.

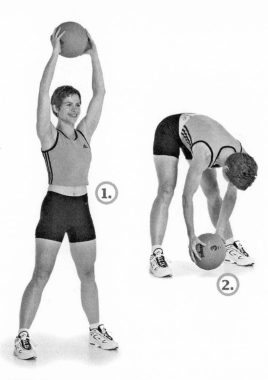

chop and twist

Muscles worked: Erector spinae, glutes, hamstrings, and obliques
Perfectly Fit bonus: Tones love-handle area
Rating: BASIC
Equipment: A medicine ball

Stand with your feet wider than shoulder-width apart and your knees slightly bent. Hold a medicine ball in both hands out in front of you, keeping your back straight and your elbows slightly bent.

In a smooth, controlled manner, bend at the waist and swing the ball down between your legs (1). Straighten back up, slowly swinging the ball over to the left (2). Then swing back down through your legs again, coming back up and twisting to the right. Continue alternating chopping and twisting from side to side in a fluid motion.

Lift Tips

○ Keep the weight light and your motion smooth and ev⌐ since this exercise uses the lower-back muscles, which tend to be weak from underuse.

○ Turn your entire body as you twist, keeping your facing in the direction of the ball.

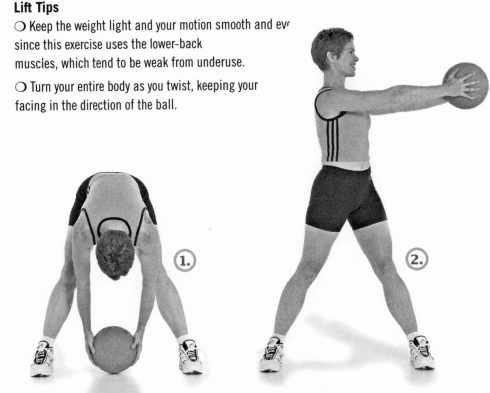

kneeling side chop

Muscles worked: Obliques, deltoids, erector spinae, and abdominals
Perfectly Fit bonus: Builds a solid trunk
Rating: BASIC
Equipment: A medicine ball

Kneel with your knees about shoulder-width apart. Hold a medicine ball in both hands over your head (1).

In a smooth, slow motion, swing the ball across your body and down to the outside of your left knee (2). Pause, then swing it back across your body to the starting position. Do one set to the left, then do one set to the right.

Lift Tips

○ Start with a light weight to get a feel for the motion and to strengthen the lower-back muscles, which tend to be weak from underuse.

○ Keep your lower body stable throughout the exercise; the motion happens from the waist up.

○ Make this exercise easier by alternating sides to start.

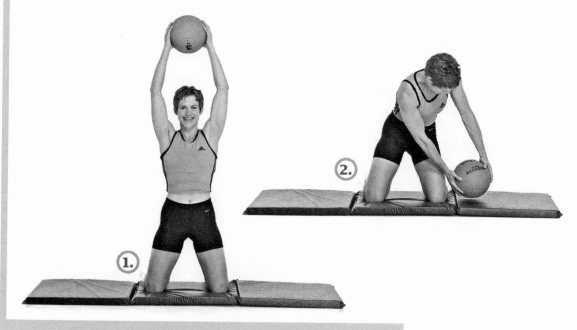

opposite arm and leg raise

Muscles worked: Rhomboids, latissimus dorsi, erector spinae, glutes, and deltoids
Perfectly Fit bonus: No more back fatigue and ache
Rating: BASIC to INTERMEDIATE
Equipment: None

Start on your hands and knees with your back straight and your head comfortably in line with your spine (1).

Simultaneously raise and straighten your left arm and your right leg so that they are extended out from your body in opposite directions and are parallel to the ground (2). Hold for 2 seconds, then slowly return to the starting position. Repeat with the opposite arm and leg.

Lift Tips

○ Keep your eyes looking down and just slightly ahead to keep your head comfortably in line with your back.

○ To make this exercise harder, add ankle weights and hold a light dumbbell in each hand.

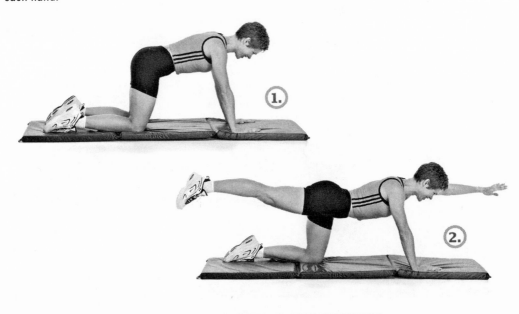

squat
and reach

Muscles worked: Hip flexors, quadriceps, hamstrings, glutes, deltoids, pectorals, and triceps
Perfectly Fit bonus: Tighter butt
Rating: INTERMEDIATE
Equipment: A medicine ball or dumbbell

Stand with your feet hip- to shoulder-width apart. Hold a medicine ball or dumbbell against your chest with both hands. Keep your elbows out to the sides.

Slowly bend at the knees and squat back as though moving your butt down toward an imaginary chair. Keep your back flat and don't allow your knees to jut over your toes. Stop when your thighs are just about parallel to the floor; don't go any lower (1). Pause, then return to the starting position. When in the "up" position, squeeze your buttocks and press the ball over your head (2). Pause, then lower it back to your chest.

Lift Tips

❍ Keep your eyes facing forward throughout the exercise; it will help you keep your back straight.

❍ Widen your stance to emphasize your hamstrings and outer thighs. Narrow it to emphasize your quads.

❍ When using a dumbbell for this exercise, hold it in front of you by its ends.

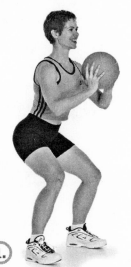

(1.)

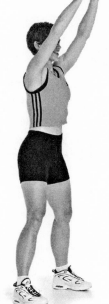

(2.)

dumbbell squat and upward press

Muscles worked: Glutes, quadriceps, hamstrings, hip flexors, triceps, and deltoids
Perfectly Fit bonus: Develops a balanced body
Rating: INTERMEDIATE
Equipment: Dumbbells

Stand with your feet shoulder-width apart and hold a dumbbell in each hand up at your shoulders, with your palms facing forward (1).

Slowly bend your knees and squat down and back. Keep your back flat, and don't allow your knees to jut over your toes or your butt to dip below knee level. At the same time, extend your arms and press the dumbbells straight over your head (2). Pause, then reverse the motion back to the starting position.

Lift Tips

○ Begin with a light weight to perfect your form.

○ Keep your eyes facing forward throughout the exercise; it will help you keep your back straight.

○ If you have a history of shoulder problems, turn the dumbbells so that your palms are facing your ears, as that reduces the chance of shoulder impingement during the exercise.

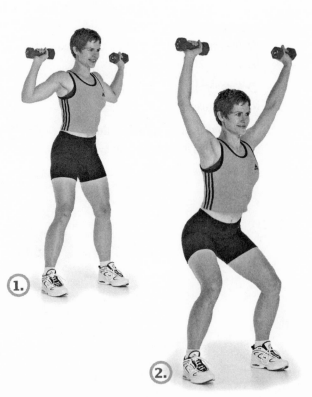

step and extend

Muscles worked: Hamstrings, hip flexors, quadriceps, glutes, adductors, deltoids, triceps, and pectorals
Perfectly Fit bonus: Sexy inner-thigh definition
Rating: INTERMEDIATE
Equipment: A medicine ball or dumbbell and an aerobic step or sturdy box

Stand about a foot away from an aerobic step or sturdy box with your feet hip-width apart. Hold a medicine ball or dumbbell in both hands against your chest (1).

Keeping your upper body straight, step forward with your left foot, placing it on the center of the step. In one motion, rise up onto the step and press the ball forward and up while extending your right leg out and back (2). Pause, then reverse the motion, stepping back down to the floor. Do one set with your left foot, then switch and repeat with your right.

Lift Tips

○ Begin with a light weight to perfect your form.

○ Make the exercise easier by alternating feet during the set.

○ When using a dumbbell for this exercise, hold it in front of you by its ends.

○ Start with just the stepping motion and add the arm motion later if you have trouble keeping your balance.

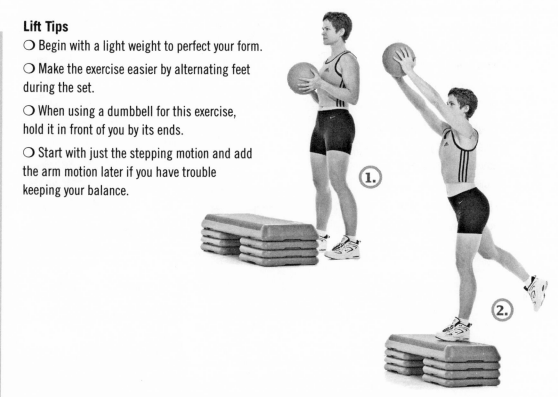

1.

2.

rising and setting sun

Muscles worked: Quadriceps, glutes, deltoids, and triceps
Perfectly Fit bonus: Tones saddlebag muscles
Rating: INTERMEDIATE
Equipment: A medicine ball

Stand with your feet in a wide straddle stance, with your toes pointed out slightly. Hold a medicine ball with both hands over your head (1).

In one move, bend your left knee and your elbows, bringing the ball down over your left thigh as you lunge in that direction (2). Your right leg should stay extended throughout the move. Do not allow your left knee to jut over your toes or your butt to dip below knee level. Pause, then, in one move, push off your left leg and extend the ball back over your head, returning to the starting position. Repeat the motion in the opposite direction without resting. The ball will move as though rising and setting over you.

Lift Tips

❍ Keep your back flat throughout the exercise; do not hunch over your knees as you squat.

❍ Make the exercise easier by holding the ball still at your chest. When you've mastered the side-to-side motion, add the overhead ball movement.

❍ Point your toes out more if you're having trouble balancing.

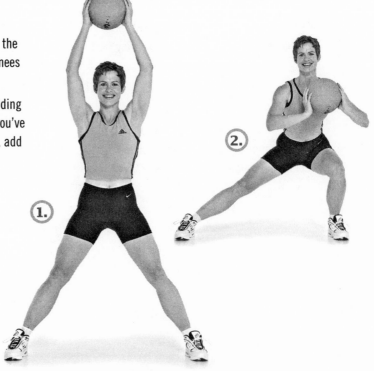

standing lunge and curl

Muscles worked: Glutes, quadriceps, hamstrings, and biceps
Perfectly Fit bonus: Better balance and flexibility
Rating: INTERMEDIATE
Equipment: Dumbbells

Stand with your left leg 2 to 3 feet in front of your right leg. Hold a pair of dumbbells down at your sides (1).

Slowly bend your left leg until your left thigh is parallel to the floor and your right leg is extended with your knee slightly bent and almost touching the floor. Be sure to keep your back straight and don't allow your left knee to jut over your toes. As you bend your leg, bend your arms and raise the weights to your chest (2). Pause, then raise yourself back up to the starting position, lowering the weights back down to your sides as you stand. Do one set, then switch and repeat with the opposite leg.

Lift Tips

○ Set aside the weights and hold on to a tabletop or chair back until you feel steady during the lunge.

○ Use lighter dumbbells than you would for regular arm curls to avoid premature arm fatigue.

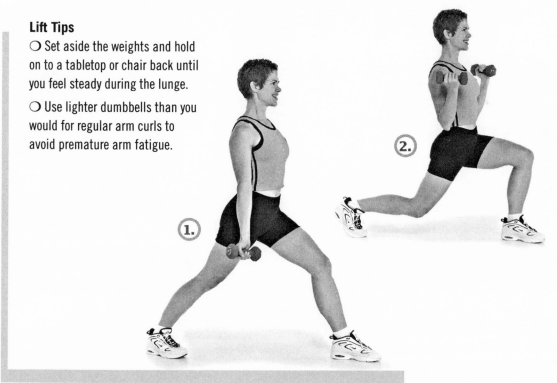

ditch digger

Muscles worked: Glutes, deltoids, quadriceps, adductors, and obliques
Perfectly Fit bonus: Tight midriff
Rating: INTERMEDIATE
Equipment: A medicine ball

Stand with your feet in a wide straddle stance, with your toes pointed out about 45 degrees. Hold a medicine ball down in front of you and keep your arms extended, your back straight, and your eyes facing forward (1).

Bend your knees about 45 degrees into a half-squat. Then, without hesitating, stand back up and swing the ball up and to the left to just above shoulder height (2). Pause, then squat again, bringing the ball back down in front of you. Stand and swing the ball to the opposite side. Alternate throughout the exercise as though digging and hoisting dirt over each shoulder.

Lift Tips

❍ Keep your motions slow and controlled to avoid overtwisting.

❍ You have swung the ball high enough when you feel the oblique on the opposite side contract to stabilize your body.

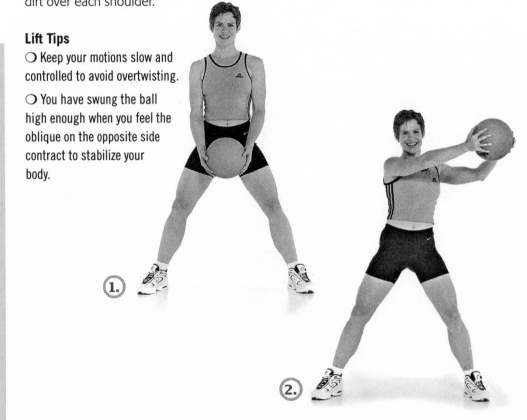

curl and half-squat

Muscles worked: Quadriceps, hamstrings, glutes, hip flexors, and biceps
Perfectly Fit bonus: Move furniture with no sweat
Rating: INTERMEDIATE
Equipment: Dumbbells

Stand with your feet shoulder-width apart. Hold a dumbbell in each hand, allowing your arms to hang down naturally at the fronts of your thighs, with your palms facing forward (1).

Slowly bend your elbows and curl the dumbbells up to your shoulders. Keeping the dumbbells close to your body and your back straight, bend your knees and slowly squat down and back about 45 degrees into a half-squat. Do not let your knees jut over your toes (2). Pause, then stand, lowering the dumbbells back to the starting position.

Lift Tips

○ Keep the weights close to your body. This will help prevent your torso from leaning forward.

○ Turn your toes out slightly to work your inner thighs more.

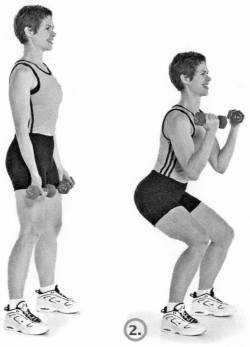

1.

2.

sprinter start

Muscles worked: Hamstrings, gastrocnemius, glutes, pectorals, and deltoids
Perfectly Fit bonus: Strong stair-climbing muscles
Rating: INTERMEDIATE
Equipment: None

Begin in a race-starting position, with your right leg forward, bent at the knee, your left leg extended straight behind your body, and your hands on the floor directly underneath your shoulders on either side of your right foot. Keep your neck straight in line with your back and your abdominals tight for balance.

Jump and switch legs, bringing the left foot forward and the right leg back, while supporting your upper body with your hands. Pause, then switch again.

Lift Tips

○ Always warm up before your routine and stretch afterward since the exercise uses quick, explosive motion.

○ Keep your head and neck straight and in line with your back throughout the exercise.

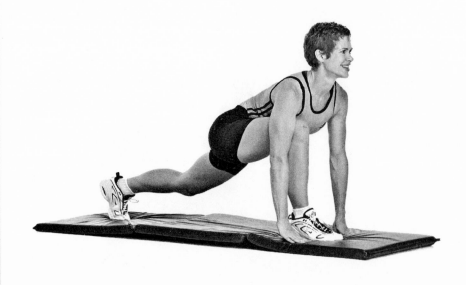

sumo squat arm raise

Muscles worked: Glutes, quadriceps, and deltoids
Perfectly Fit bonus: Firm ballerina butt
Rating: INTERMEDIATE
Equipment: Dumbbells

Stand with your feet in a wide straddle stance with your toes pointed out 45 degrees or more. Hold a dumbbell in each hand, allowing your arms to hang down naturally at your sides, with your palms facing in (1).

All in one move, slowly raise your arms up and out to the sides, keeping your elbows slightly bent, until your arms reach shoulder level and your palms are facing the floor, and bend your knees and lower your body until your thighs are almost parallel to the floor. Do not allow your knees to jut over your toes and your butt to dip lower than your knees (2). Pause, then return to the starting position.

Lift Tips

○ Use light weights since the exercise puts a lot of demand on small muscles.

○ Keep your head in line with your back to prevent neck strain.

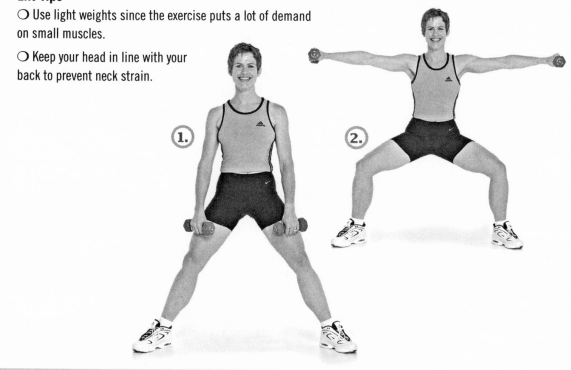

synchronized kickback

Muscles worked: Glutes and triceps
Perfectly Fit bonus: No more jiggly arms
Rating: INTERMEDIATE
Equipment: A tabletop or sturdy chair and a dumbbell

Wearing ankle weights, place your left hand on a tabletop or chair back for balance. Bend forward slightly from the waist, keeping your back flat. Grasp a dumbbell in your right hand and let your arm hang down naturally.

Bend your right arm and lift the weight up toward your chest while bending your right knee and lifting your leg slightly (1). Then, in one motion, straighten your right arm, bringing the weight behind you; tighten your buttock; and extend your right leg behind you. Keep your head, neck, and back aligned (2). Hold for 2 seconds. Do one set with your right hand and leg, then switch and repeat with your left hand and leg.

Lift Tips

○ Stand up straight instead of bending forward to keep your back from getting fatigued.

○ Make the leg portion easier by eliminating the ankle weights.

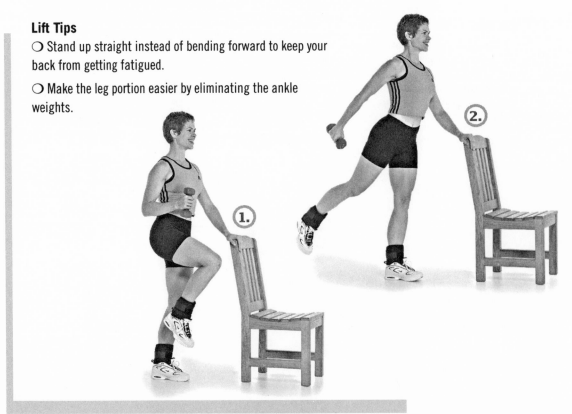

ball swing knee kick

Muscles worked: Quadriceps, hamstrings, glutes, deltoids, obliques, and abdominals
Perfectly Fit bonus: A taut, balanced body
Rating: INTERMEDIATE to ADVANCED
Equipment: A medicine ball

Stand with your left leg 2 to 3 feet in front of your right leg, with your left foot flat on the floor and your right foot balanced on the ball of the foot. Hold a medicine ball up and out in front of you (1).

In one smooth motion, swing your right knee forward and up while swinging the ball down and to the right, so that it ends up on the outside of your right thigh (2). Swing back to the starting position, pressing the ball back up and extending your right leg back. Do one set with your right leg, then switch and repeat with your left.

Lift Tips

○ Turn your head in the direction of the ball as you bring it down for added oblique work.

○ Perform this exercise in a slow, controlled manner to get the best results.

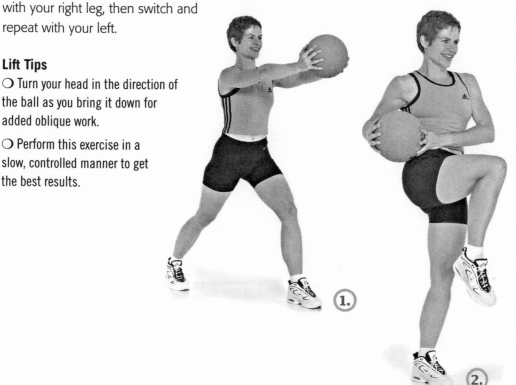

1.

2.

lunge row

Muscles worked: Quadriceps, glutes, pectorals, hip flexors, deltoids, and rhomboids
Perfectly Fit bonus: Great agility
Rating: INTERMEDIATE TO ADVANCED
Equipment: Dumbbells

Stand with your left leg 2 to 3 feet in front of your right leg. Hold a pair of dumbbells out in front of you with your palms down and weights horizontal to the floor (1).

Slowly bend your left leg and lower your torso toward your left knee. Be sure to keep your back straight and do not allow your left knee to jut over your toes. At the same time, squeeze your shoulder blades together and row the dumbbells back toward your body so they end up at either side of your chest (2). Pause, then return to the starting position. Finish one set, then switch and repeat with the right leg.

Lift Tips

○ Use light weights since this exercise puts a fair amount of tension on your shoulders.

○ Make the exercise easier by turning your palms so they face each other and the weights are vertical to your body throughout the exercise.

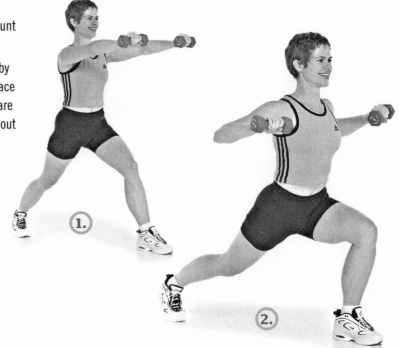

lift, curl, and reach

Muscles worked: Glutes, quadriceps, hamstrings, hip flexors, biceps, triceps, and deltoids
Perfectly Fit bonus: Makes putting away heavy groceries a breeze
Rating: ADVANCED
Equipment: A medicine ball

Stand with your feet slightly wider than shoulder-width apart and place a medicine ball an arm's distance away on the floor in front of you.

Slowly bend at the knees and squat down and back. Keep your back flat, and don't allow your knees to jut over your toes or your butt to dip below knee level. Bend forward slightly, extend your arms, and pick up the ball (1). Slowly stand back up, curling the ball to your chest as you do (2). When you reach the standing position, press the ball over your head, keeping your knees slightly bent (3). Pause, then bring the ball back to your chest. Extend your arms forward and squat again, placing the ball back on the ground.

Lift Tips
❍ Keep your eyes facing forward throughout exercise; it will help you keep your back straight.

❍ Begin with a light weight to perfect your form.

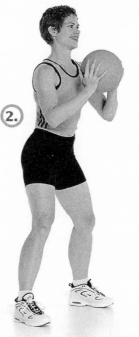

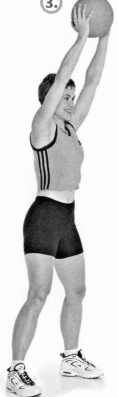

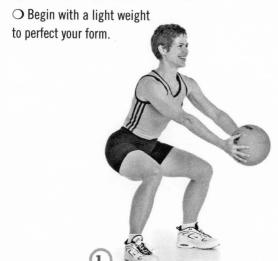

Upper Body

The following exercises are considered upper-body compound moves because you must use two or more major muscles in your upper body to perform them correctly.

dumbbell press

Muscles worked: Pectorals, triceps, and deltoids
Perfectly Fit bonus: Killer cleavage
Rating: BASIC
Equipment: An optional aerobic step or bench and dumbbells

Lie on your back on an aerobic step or bench (the floor is fine if neither is available) with your feet flat on the floor or on the bench if that is more comfortable. Hold the dumbbells lined up end to end (but not touching) over your chest with your arms extended, your knuckles facing the ceiling, and your thumbs facing each other (1).

Slowly lower the weights so that your elbows point down and out perpendicular to your body. Stop when the weights are about even with your chest (2). (If you're on the floor, your arms will be on the floor.) Slowly return to the starting position.

Lift Tips

○ Keep your spine steady and your back flat and supported throughout the exercise; do not arch your back or lift your hips.

○ Concentrate on contracting and squeezing your chest muscles to lift the weight for maximum effectiveness.

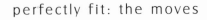

upright row

Muscles worked: Deltoids, trapezius, and forearms
Perfectly Fit bonus: Hoist groceries with ease
Rating: BASIC
Equipment: Dumbbells

Stand with your legs about shoulder-width apart with your knees slightly bent. Hold a dumbbell in each hand and let your arms hang down at the fronts of your thighs with your palms facing your legs (1).

Squeeze your shoulder blades, bend your elbows, and pull the weights up and out to the sides until your elbows reach about shoulder height (2). Pause, then straighten your arms and lower the weights back to the starting position.

Lift Tips

○ Keep your shoulders down throughout the exercise; do not allow them to shrug up toward your ears.

○ Hold your head straight and in line with your spine; do not tilt it back or jut your chin forward.

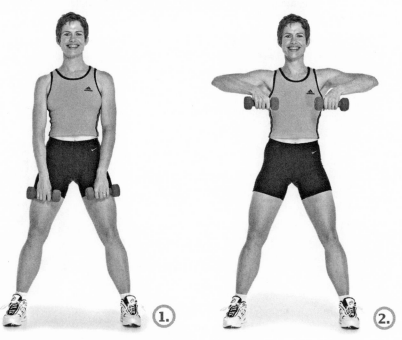

seated
back fly

Muscles worked: Rhomboids, deltoids, and triceps
Perfectly Fit bonus: A mean backhand on the tennis court
Rating: BASIC
Equipment: A bench or sturdy chair and dumbbells

Sit on the edge of a bench
or a sturdy chair with your feet together flat on the floor. Hold a dumbbell in each hand. Keeping your back flat, bend at the waist and lower
your chest toward your knees. Let your arms hang down on either side
of your legs with your hands by your knees (1).

Squeeze your shoulder blades and raise the weights out to the sides,
keeping your elbows slightly bent, until your arms are outstretched parallel to the floor (2). Pause, then slowly lower the weights back to the
starting position.

Lift Tips

○ Keep your head in line with your spine throughout the exercise.

○ Keep your abdominal muscles contracted for support throughout the movement.

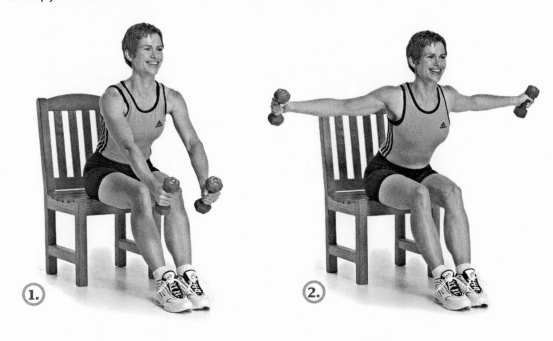

lying overhead pullover

Muscles worked: Pectorals, latissimus dorsi, deltoids, and triceps
Perfectly Fit bonus: Stretches tight, shortened chest muscles to improve posture
Rating: BASIC
Equipment: An optional aerobic step or bench and a medicine ball or dumbbell

Lie on your back on an aerobic step or bench (the floor is fine if neither is available, but the exercise will be less effective). Keep your back flat on the bench, with your feet flat on the floor or on the bench if that is more comfortable. Hold a medicine ball or dumbbell in both hands with your arms extended straight over your chest. Keep your elbows slightly bent (1).

Slowly lower the weight straight back over your head until your arms are parallel to the floor, or as far as is comfortably possible (2). Pause, then slowly raise the weight back to the starting position. Do not arch your back.

Lift Tips

❍ Use a light weight until you get comfortable with the motion.

❍ When using a dumbbell for this exercise, hold it by an end so that your hands wrap around one of the bells.

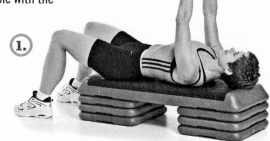

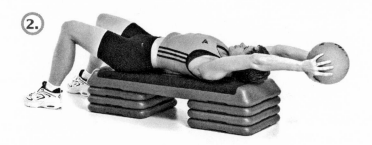

pushup

Muscles worked: Pectorals, triceps, and deltoids
Perfectly Fit bonus: Gives your ego a boost
Rating: BASIC to ADVANCED
Equipment: None

Start on your hands and knees, with your hips extended so that your body forms a straight line from your head to your knees. Cross your ankles for stability (1). Your hands should be in line with your shoulders.

Bend your elbows and slowly lower your torso toward the floor (2). Stop when your shoulders are in line with your elbows, then push up.

Lift Tips

○ Keep your shoulders down in their natural position as you lift and lower your torso; do not let them shrug up toward your ears.

○ Make this exercise more challenging by performing it on your toes rather than on your knees.

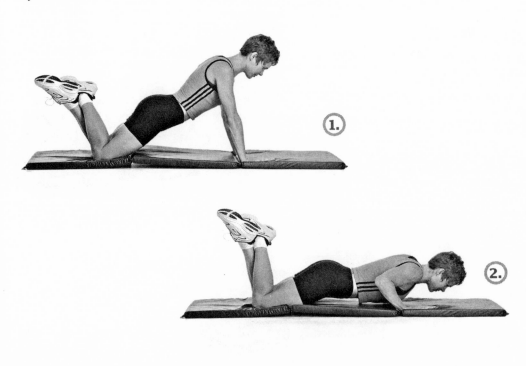

arm raise pullover

Muscles worked: Latissimus dorsi, triceps, pectorals, and deltoids
Perfectly Fit bonus: Strong, limber shoulders
Rating: INTERMEDIATE
Equipment: An optional aerobic step or bench and dumbbells

Lie on your back on an aerobic step or bench (the floor is fine if neither is available, but the exercise will be less effective) with your feet flat on the floor or on the bench if that is more comfortable. Hold a dumbbell in each hand, allowing your arms to hang down naturally at your sides, with your palms facing down (1).

Raise your arms straight up and over your chest so that the dumbbells touch end to end, with your palms facing up. Keeping the dumbbells together, slowly lower your arms back over your head until they are straight out behind you (2). Pause, then slowly reverse the motion, bringing the dumbbells back over your head and above your chest, then lowering them to your sides.

Lift Tips
○ Keep your spine steady and your back flat and supported throughout the exercise; do not arch your back or lift your hips.

○ Use light weights since this exercise works the small rotator cuff muscles.

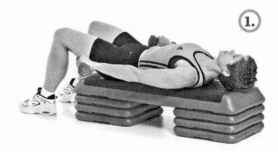

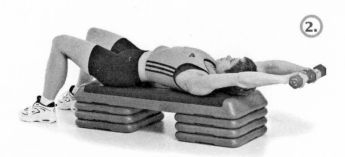

curl and press

Muscles worked: Biceps, triceps, deltoids, and trapezius
Perfectly Fit bonus: Kissably curvy nape
Rating: INTERMEDIATE
Equipment: A sturdy chair and dumbbells

Sit on a sturdy chair with your feet flat on the floor comfortably in front of you. Hold a dumbbell in each hand with your arms extended down to your sides and your palms facing forward.

Keeping your upper body stable, bend your elbows and curl the weights up toward your shoulders (1). Without hesitating, rotate your wrists so that your palms are facing out in front of you. Press the weights over your head (2). Pause, then slowly reverse the motion, lowering the weights to your shoulders, rotating your palms in toward your body, and lowering the weights back down to your sides.

Lift Tips

○ Maintain upright posture throughout the exercise, keeping your back straight and your eyes forward.

○ Keep your shoulders down as you curl and lift; do not allow them to shrug up toward your ears.

○ Sit back in the chair if you need more support.

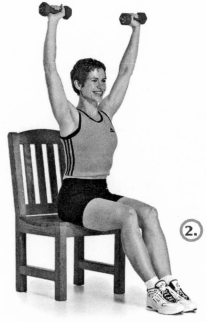

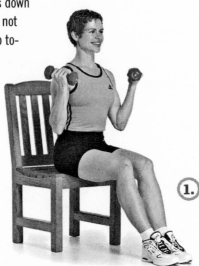

curl
and punch

Muscles worked: Biceps, triceps, and deltoids
Perfectly Fit bonus: Sleek, rounded shoulders
Rating: INTERMEDIATE
Equipment: Dumbbells

Stand with your feet shoulder-width apart. Hold a dumbbell in each hand, allowing your arms to hang down naturally at your sides, with your palms facing forward.

Slowly bend your left elbow, bringing the weight up toward your left shoulder (1). Without hesitating, rotate your wrist so your palm is facing away from you, then extend your straight arm out directly in front of you in a punching motion (2). Pause, then reverse the motion, bringing the weight back to your shoulder, rotating your wrist as you do, so that your palm is facing your body. Lower the weight back to the starting position. Repeat with your right arm. Alternate arms throughout the set.

Lift Tips

○ Keep your body stable by bending your knees slightly throughout the exercise.

○ Perform the exercise in a slow and controlled manner. Do not "throw" a fast punch and do not lock your elbows during the outward extension.

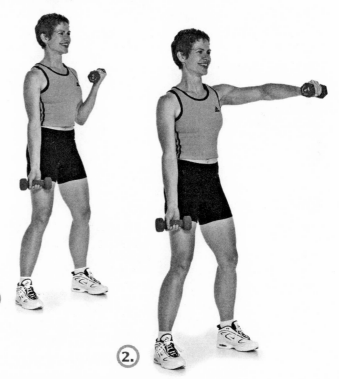

1.

2.

seated row

Muscles worked: Trapezius, latissimus dorsi, rhomboids, and biceps
Perfectly Fit bonus: Curvy, sexy back
Rating: INTERMEDIATE
Equipment: A sturdy chair or bench and dumbbells

Sit on the edge of a sturdy chair or a bench, with your knees bent about 45 degrees, so that your feet are out in front of your knees. Hold a dumbbell in each hand. Keeping your back straight, lean forward slightly and extend your arms down at an angle in front of you, so that the weights are on either side of your knees and your palms are facing in (1).

Squeezing your shoulder blades together, bend your arms and pull your elbows back, bringing the weights up to your hips and waist (2). Pause, then slowly lower the weights to the starting position.

Lift Tips

○ Keep your elbows close to your body throughout the entire exercise; do not allow them to jut out to the sides.

○ Make this exercise less stressful on your shoulders by substituting an exercise band for the dumbbells. Simply sit in the same position and loop an exercise band around the balls of your feet. Hold an end in each hand and simulate the rowing motion by pulling the band ends.

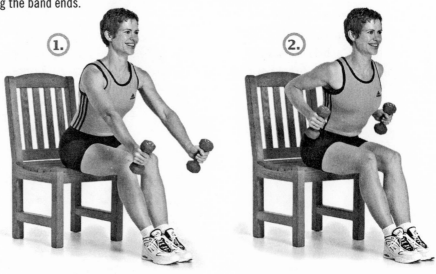

ball press and ab curl

Muscles worked: Pectorals, triceps, and abdominals
Perfectly Fit bonus: A tighter tummy
Rating: INTERMEDIATE
Equipment: A medicine ball or dumbbells

Lie on your back on the floor with your feet flat on the floor and your knees bent at a 90-degree angle. Holding a medicine ball or dumbbells with both hands, let the weight rest lightly on your chest, keeping your elbows out to the sides. Tilt your pelvis slightly to keep your back flat against the floor (1).

All in one move, contract your chest muscles and straighten your elbows, pushing the ball straight up above your chest. Keeping your arms outstretched and stable, immediately lift your head and shoulders off the floor about 30 degrees (2). Hold for 2 seconds. In one motion, lower the ball back to your body and lower your body to the floor.

Lift Tips

○ Keep your head and neck aligned throughout the exercise; do not jut your head forward or crane your neck.

○ If you substitute dumbbells in this exercise, use light weights and keep them together end to end throughout the entire exercise.

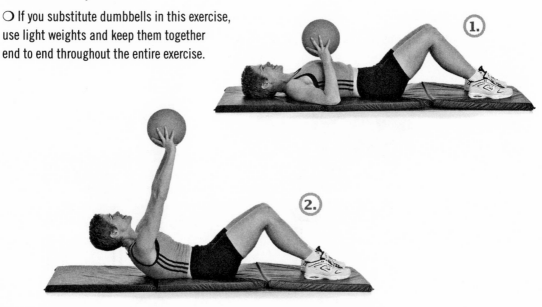

row and kickback

Muscles worked: Rhomboids, latissimus dorsi, trapezius, and triceps
Perfectly Fit bonus: Open heavy doors with ease
Rating: INTERMEDIATE
Equipment: A dumbbell and a sturdy chair or bench

Hold a dumbbell in your right hand, with your palm facing in. Rest your left knee and left hand on a chair seat or bench for support. Place your right foot on the floor, with your knee slightly bent. Keep your back straight and flat and your head down in a straight line with your back. Let the arm holding the weight hang down toward the floor.

Slowly pull the weight up to your chest (1). Your right elbow should be pointing toward the ceiling as you lift. Hold for 1 second, then extend your arm behind your body so that your entire arm is parallel to the floor (2). Pause, then reverse the motion, bending your elbow and slowly lowering the weight toward the floor. Do one set with your right arm, then switch and repeat with your left.

Lift Tips

○ Keep your back flat and your eyes facing down throughout the exercise.

○ Keep your arm close to your body as you lift, extend, and lower the weight.

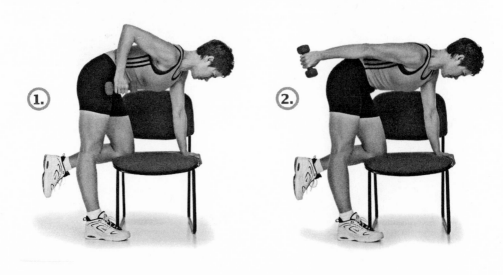

engine pull

Muscles worked: Rhomboids, trapezius, and triceps
Perfectly Fit bonus: Shopping bag stamina
Rating: INTERMEDIATE
Equipment: A dumbbell

Stand with your left leg 2 to 3 feet in front of your right leg, with your feet facing forward. Keeping your back straight, bend your left knee, lean slightly forward, and place your left hand on your thigh for support. Hold a dumbbell in your right hand, allowing it to hang down to the inside of your left knee, with your palm facing in (1).

Pull your right arm out and back to the right, leading with your elbow. Stop when you feel the back of your shoulder and the middle of your shoulder blades tighten (2). The weight will be at about chest level or beyond. Pause, then return to the starting position. The motion is similar to pulling a cord on a boat engine or a lawn mower, hence the name. Do one set with your right arm, then switch and repeat with your left.

Lift Tips

❍ Keep the motion slow and controlled, not jerky or explosive, even though it mimics a pulling motion.

❍ Resist the urge to let your shoulders ride up during the exercise. Keep them down and relaxed.

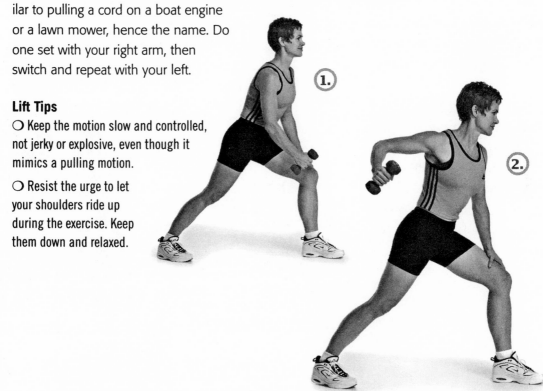

angel wings

Muscles worked: Biceps, triceps, and deltoids
Perfectly Fit bonus: Tireless waving and cheering at the next game
Rating: INTERMEDIATE to ADVANCED
Equipment: A sturdy chair or bench and dumbbells

Sit on the edge of a chair or bench with your feet flat on the floor. Hold a dumbbell in each hand, with your arms extended down at your sides and your palms facing forward (1).

Slowly bend your elbows and curl the dumbbells up toward your shoulders, rotating your wrists as you lift, so that your palms end up facing each other. Without hesitating, raise the weights over your head until your arms are almost completely straight. Rotate your wrists so that your palms face outward (2). While your arms are still straight, lower the weights out to your sides and back down to the starting position.

Lift Tips

○ Use lighter weights than usual since this exercise uses small shoulder muscles and connective tissue.

○ Keep your shoulders down and relaxed during the exercise; do not allow them to shrug up toward your ears.

○ Do not lock your elbows at any point during the exercise; keep them slightly soft for support.

○ Sit back on the chair if you need more support.

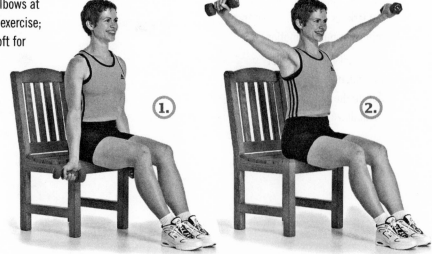

pullup

Muscles worked: Rhomboids, trapezius, latissimus dorsi, pectorals, biceps, triceps, and forearms
Perfectly Fit bonus: Feel like Superwoman
Rating: ADVANCED
Equipment: A pullup bar or a very sturdy table

Grasp a pullup bar (most workout facilities have one), using an underhand grip so that your palms are facing in and your arms are slightly more than shoulder-width apart. Hang from the bar with your knees slightly bent and your ankles crossed.

Using your arm and back muscles, slowly pull yourself up until your chin is above the level of the bar. Pause, then lower yourself back to the starting position.

To do this at home without a pullup bar, lie on your back beneath a *sturdy* table with your knees bent and your feet flat on the floor. Reach up and grasp the edge of the table so that you're suspended from the ground (1). Slowly bend your elbows and pull your torso up until your chin is above the level of the tabletop (2). Pause, then lower yourself back to the starting position. Keep your back straight throughout the exercise.

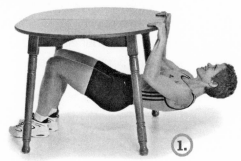

Be sure that the table you use is very sturdy and stable. You may also want to ask a friend to spot you the first few times you do this exercise.

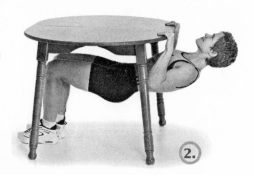

Lift Tips

○ This is an especially difficult exercise for many women, as we have less upper-body strength than men. But it's a big kick when you can finally do a few. If you can't manage even one when you start, don't sweat it. Just come back and try again periodically as you become stronger.

○ If you have enough strength to pull yourself up a few inches but can't make it all the way to the bar or table, have a friend help lift you up, then lower yourself slowly. Soon you'll be doing the whole pullup on your own.

chair dip

Muscles worked: Triceps, lower pectorals, and deltoids
Perfectly Fit bonus: Supersexy arms
Rating: ADVANCED
Equipment: A sturdy chair

Brace a sturdy chair against a wall so it won't move. Sit on the edge of the chair and grasp the seat of the chair with both hands on either side of your butt. Extend your legs straight out in front of you and inch your butt off the edge of the chair, keeping your arms extended and supporting your weight with the heels of your hands (1).

Bend your elbows back, and keeping your body close to the chair, smoothly dip down a few inches, or until your shoulders are in line with your elbows (2). Push yourself back to the starting position.

Lift Tips

○ Keep your shoulders down throughout the exercise; do not let them shrug up toward your ears.

○ Make the exercise easier by keeping one knee bent and extending only one leg.

① .

② .

Lower Body

The following exercises are considered lower–body compound moves because you must use two or more major muscles in your lower body to perform them correctly.

forward and back kick

Muscles worked: Quadriceps, hamstrings, hip flexors, and glutes
Perfectly Fit bonus: Bound up the stairs
Rating: BASIC
Equipment: Ankle weights and a sturdy chair

Wearing ankle weights, stand to the left of a chair with your feet hip-width apart and your toes forward. Rest your left hand on the back of the chair for support.

Slowly lift your right knee until your right thigh is parallel to the ground (1). Lower it and slowly swing your right leg back behind you until it is fully extended (2). Do one set with your right leg, then switch and repeat with your left.

Lift Tips

❍ Begin with a light weight to perfect your form.

❍ Keep your back straight and your eyes facing forward throughout the exercise; do not lean forward or backward as you move your legs.

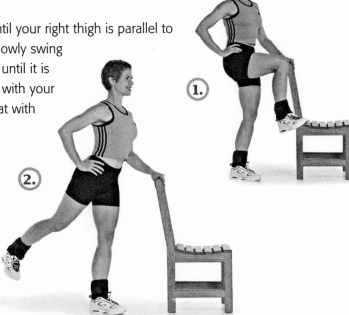

side to side

Muscles worked: Quadriceps, abductors, adductors, hamstrings, and glutes
Perfectly Fit bonus: Lengthens and limbers tight groin muscles
Rating: BASIC
Equipment: Dumbbells

Stand with your legs shoulder-width apart with your toes pointed out about 45 degrees and your back flat and straight. Hold a dumbbell in each hand and rest them at your hips (1).

Take a giant step to the left and bend your left knee until your thigh is parallel to the floor, keeping your right leg extended. Do not allow your left knee to jut over your toes or your butt to dip below your knee (2). Pause, then return to the starting position and repeat the motion to the right side without resting.

Lift Tips

❍ To make this exercise easier, try it first without weights, holding your hands on your hips.

❍ To make it more difficult, hold the dumbbells up at your shoulders while performing the exercise.

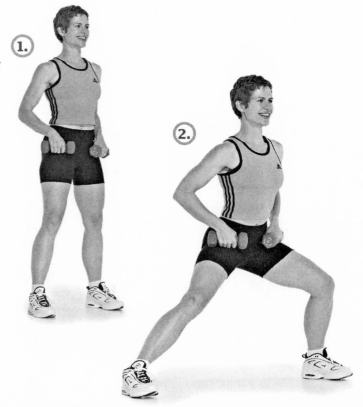

step and heel raise

Muscles worked: Hamstrings, quadriceps, hip flexors, glutes, adductors, and gastrocnemius
Perfectly Fit bonus: Skirt-sexy calves
Rating: BASIC to ADVANCED
Equipment: An aerobic step

Stand about a foot away from a step with your feet hip-width apart and your right hand on your hip. Hold on to a wall or banister with your left arm for support if needed, or put both hands on hips.

Keeping your upper body straight, step forward with your left foot, placing it on the center of the step. Straighten your left leg, lifting your right foot off the floor. Squeeze your buttocks and extend your right leg behind you, with your toes pointed toward the floor (1). Pause, then raise your body up on the ball of your left foot (2). Hold for 1 second. Reverse the motion, lowering yourself onto your left foot, bringing your right leg down, and stepping back to the floor. Repeat with the opposite leg. Alternate legs throughout the exercise.

Lift Tips
○ Keep your back straight and flat and your eyes facing forward throughout the entire exercise.

○ Make the exercise more challenging by placing your hands on your hips throughout the exercise.

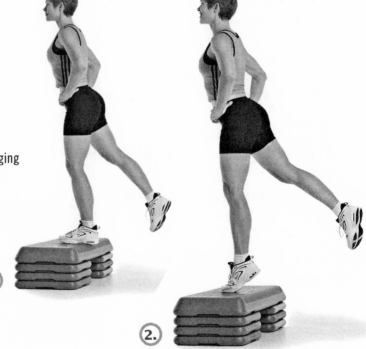

1.

2.

duck squat toe raise

Muscles worked: Glutes, quadriceps, adductors, and gastrocnemius
Perfectly Fit bonus: Dancer's legs
Rating: INTERMEDIATE
Equipment: A medicine ball or dumbbell

Stand with your feet wider than shoulder-width apart and your toes pointing out about 45 degrees. Hold a medicine ball or dumbbell in both hands, extending your arms straight down in front of your body.

Slowly bend your knees and lower your body until your thighs are parallel to the floor. Do not allow your knees to jut over your toes or your butt to dip below knee level (1). Immediately, raise your heels and stand up on the balls of your feet (2). Hold for 1 second, then lower your heels and raise yourself back to the starting position.

Lift Tips

○ Keep your back straight and your shoulders down throughout the exercise. Leaning forward slightly from the waist is natural.

○ Take out the toe-raise step until you are comfortable with the squat. This will make the exercise easier.

○ When using a dumbbell for this exercise, hold it by an end so that your hands wrap around one of the bells.

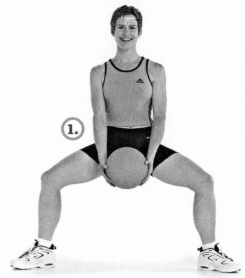

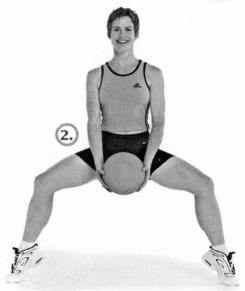

rockette

Muscles worked: Glutes and quadriceps
Perfectly Fit bonus: Strong knee-supporting muscles
Rating: INTERMEDIATE
Equipment: A sturdy chair

Wearing ankle weights, stand with your feet hip-width apart and your toes pointed straight ahead. Hold on to the back of a chair for balance and support.

Slowly swing your right knee up so that your right thigh and the bottom of your right foot are parallel to the floor (1). Pause, then extend your right leg so that it extends out straight from your body (2). Pause again, then reverse the motion, bending your right knee and lowering the leg back to the floor. Do one set with your right leg, then switch and repeat with your left.

Lift Tips

❍ Make the exercise easier by alternating legs throughout the exercise.

❍ Make the exercise easier by eliminating the ankle weights.

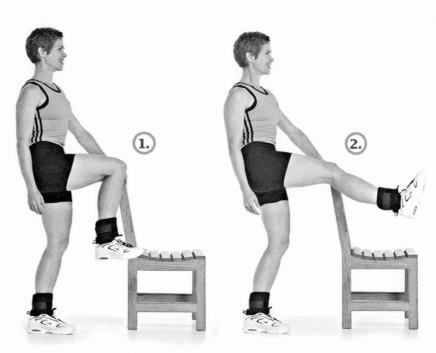

squat and side lift

Muscles worked: Glutes, hamstrings, quadriceps, hip flexors, and abductors
Perfectly Fit bonus: Tight, toned outside cheeks
Rating: INTERMEDIATE
Equipment: Ankle weights

Wearing ankle weights, stand with your feet shoulder-width apart, with your hands on your hips, your elbows out to the sides, and your toes slightly pointed out.

Slowly bend at the knees and squat back as though moving your butt down toward an imaginary chair. Keep your back flat, and don't allow your knees to jut over your toes. Stop when your thighs are just about parallel to the floor; don't go any lower (1). Pause, then straighten your legs, lifting your left leg off the floor and out to the side as you stand (2). Pause again, then return to the starting position. Repeat, lifting your right leg to the side this time. Alternate legs throughout the exercise.

Lift Tips

○ Keep your head straight and your eyes facing forward throughout the exercise.

○ To make the exercise harder, hold a light dumbbell in each hand.

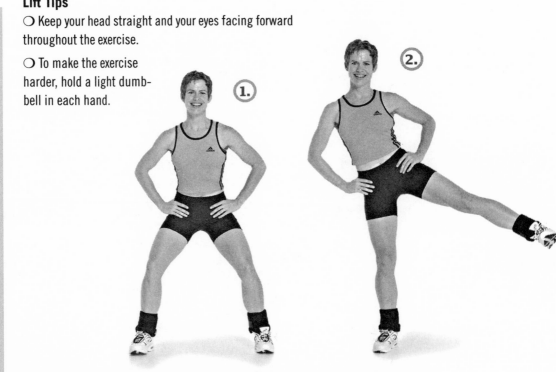

side step and squat

Muscles worked: Glutes, abductors, quadriceps, and hamstrings
Perfectly Fit bonus: No more droopy lower butt
Rating: INTERMEDIATE to ADVANCED
Equipment: An aerobic step or bench

With your feet hip- to shoulder-width apart and toes pointing forward, stand with an aerobic step or bench 2 feet to your right. Hold your hands on your hips for support (1).

Slowly step up to the side with your right foot, placing your foot squarely on the step. With your right foot on the step and your left foot on the floor, slowly bend both knees and squat back as though sitting on a chair. Keep your weight back and do not allow your knees to jut over your toes or your butt to dip below knee level (2). Pause, then straighten your legs and bring your right foot back down to the ground. Do one set with your right foot, then switch and repeat with your left.

Lift Tips

○ Keep your upper body straight and stable throughout the exercise. Leaning forward slightly from the waist is natural.

○ To make it more challenging, hold dumbbells at your hips throughout the exercise.

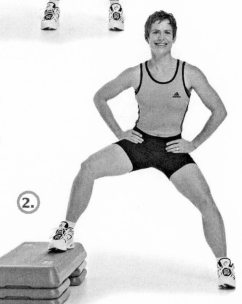

one-legged lunge

Muscles worked: Glutes, quadriceps, and hamstrings
Perfectly Fit bonus: Drop-dead legs
Rating: ADVANCED
Equipment: A sturdy chair or bench

Stand about 2 feet in front of a sturdy chair or bench with your back to it. Bend your left knee and extend your left leg behind you, putting the top of your left foot on the seat of the chair. Keep your back straight, your head aligned with your spine, and your eyes facing forward (1).

Slowly bend your right knee until it is parallel to the floor. Do not allow your right knee to jut over your toes (2). Pause, then rise back to the starting position. Do one set with your right leg, then switch and repeat with your left.

Lift Tips

○ Practice doing regular lunges before trying this exercise since this is a tough move.

○ Make this move more challenging by holding dumbbells down at your sides.

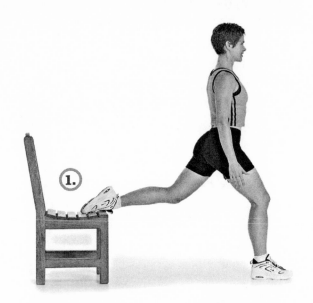

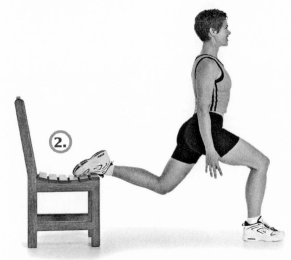

PERFECTLY FIT GOAL:
shapely, strong arms

The first sign of a fabulous body

Just a few years ago, most women were arm-phobic when it came to strength training. "I don't want big muscles on my arms!" would be the first words out of their mouths when I tried to sell them on working with weights.

That's all changed. Naturally, women still don't want steroid-freak upper-body bulk. But thanks to celebs like Madonna who have arms to die for, women are finally seeing the benefits of biceps. Today, trainers field dozens of questions from women who want to know how to shape up their arms first and their thighs second.

Sleeveless and Sexy

The main reason strong, toned arms are such a big deal for women is that like hips and thighs, the back of the upper arm is a spot where women typically store fat. Left unchecked, this fat storage can give you that jiggly "matronly" appearance most women hate. Fortunately, this problem spot is a pretty quick fix. Since you have proportionately less fat on your arms than you do on your legs, and it's less "stubborn," your arms respond more quickly to exercise and you see results sooner.

Just in case you're still concerned: Lifting weights will *not* give you manly arms. Yes, your biceps and triceps will grow a little, but only to give you firm, toned arms that'll turn heads when you wear tank tops. Even better: Strong arms make for independent women who can lift packages, hang wall art, and open stubborn jars all on their own.

The following exercises are designed to isolate specific muscles in the arms, such as the biceps, triceps, forearms, and the deltoids, to create sundress-shapely muscle tone. Some of these moves may be new to you, while others are classic, very effective moves that deserve a spot in any good training routine.

Getting started. If you're brand new to weight training, choose two or more of these exercises (one for your biceps, one for your triceps, and one for your shoulders) to incorporate into a full-body routine, like you'll find in part 3. If you already work out but want stronger, shapelier arms, tack on a few of these exercises to your existing routine. Start with one set of 10 to 12 repetitions and work up to two sets of 12 to 15 reps. Rest for 20 seconds between sets. See "Exercise Ratings"

PERFECTLY FIT TIP

Tone your arms by curling everyday items around the house, such as soup cans for biceps curls. These mini-workouts complement your regular routine and help keep your muscles strong.

between
YOU&ME

Arm exercises are by far the most immediately satisfying. Arms shape up quickly, and you see them often in day-to-day life, so you have a constant reminder that your hard work is paying off.

on page 48 to determine which level of exercise is best for you.

What to expect. Most of these exercises are fairly straightforward and don't require much balance or coordination to be performed correctly. They might be a little tough muscle-wise, however, especially the triceps exercises. Even though we use our biceps all the time for hefting shopping bags, briefcases, and babies, we don't use our little triceps muscles quite so often. Start with a light, manageable weight for those exercises.

Safety first. The farther you hold a weight out from your body, the harder it becomes to lift. Always start with a light weight when doing exercises that emphasize shoulder muscles. That will keep you from putting too much stress on your rotator cuff muscles and the connective tissues surrounding your shoulder joint. Also, keep your upper body still when doing arm exercises; avoid swaying back and forth to assist with the lift.

Results. Perform your arm exercises 2 or 3 days a week (just not on consecutive days; your muscles need a rest), and you'll feel stronger in just 2 weeks. After 3 to 4 weeks, you'll start seeing results.

Beautiful Biceps

The following exercises are designed to strengthen and tone the muscles in the fronts of your upper arms. As a bonus, you'll find that chores that once felt tough, such as loading groceries into your car or carrying boxes to the attic, will be a breeze.

simultaneous dumbbell curl

Rating: BASIC
Equipment: Dumbbells

Stand with your feet shoulder-width apart and your knees slightly bent for support. Hold a dumbbell in each hand with your palms facing out (1).

Slowly curl the dumbbells up toward your collarbone (2). Pause, then slowly lower the weights back to the starting position.

Lift Tips

❍ Keep your upper arms and elbows close to your body throughout the exercise to really focus on your biceps.

❍ Make the exercise a little easier by sitting on the edge of a chair instead of standing.

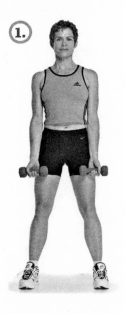

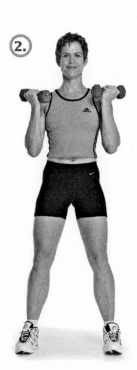

concentration curl

Rating: BASIC TO INTERMEDIATE

Equipment: A sturdy chair or bench and dumbbells

Sit on a bench or the edge of a chair with your legs apart. Hold a weight in your right hand. Bend slightly from the waist (keeping your back straight) and let your right arm hang down with your right elbow resting against the inside of your right thigh. Place your left forearm across the top of your legs for support (1).

Slowly bend your right elbow, curling the weight toward your right shoulder (2). Pause at the top of the lift. Slowly lower the weight back to the starting position. Complete one set with your right arm, then repeat with your left.

Lift Tips

○ Be careful not to swing the weight during this exercise, or you'll do your biceps little good. Lift and lower slowly.

○ Keep your upper body perfectly still while you curl your arm. If you need to use your back or torso to assist you, the weight is too heavy.

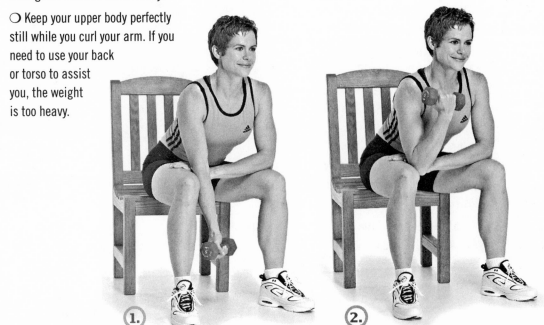

1.   2.

Taut Triceps

The following exercises are designed to strengthen and tone those underworked little muscles on the backs of your upper arms. Well-toned triceps not only give your arms that sexy curve along the back but they also make it much easier to push open heavy doors and to throw a knockout punch in your cardio kickboxing class.

behind-your-back arm raise

Rating: BASIC
Equipment: Dumbbells

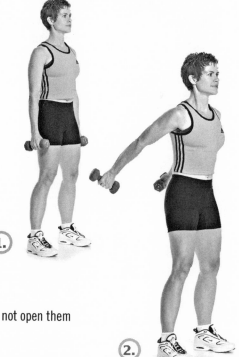

Stand with your feet about hip-width apart and your knees slightly bent for support. Hold a dumbbell in each hand, allowing your arms to hang naturally at your sides with your palms facing in (1).

Keeping your arms straight, slowly raise your arms behind you as high as comfortably possible (2). (Your palms may turn slightly up.) Hold for a moment, then slowly lower your arms back to the starting position.

Lift Tips

○ Stand tall throughout the exercise. Do not lean forward or arch your back.

○ Try to raise your arms directly behind you while lifting; do not open them out to the sides.

french curl

Lie on an aerobic step or
on the floor with a supportive pillow beneath your head, shoulders, and
upper back. Bend your knees 90 degrees and place your feet flat on
the floor. Hold a pair of dumbbells straight up above your body, angled
slightly back, so that your fists are above your head and your palms are
facing each other (1).

Keeping the rest of your body still, slowly bend your elbows and
lower the weights behind your head (2). Pause, then straighten your elbows and return to the starting position.

Lift Tips

○ Always start with a light weight to get
comfortable with the movement.

○ Your upper arms and elbows should remain
in the same position throughout the exercise;
don't allow your arms to move forward and
back.

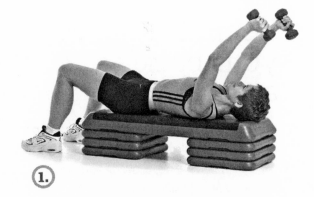

1.

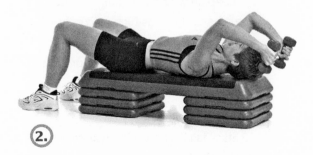

2.

lying cross-body triceps extension

Rating: INTERMEDIATE to ADVANCED
Equipment: An optional aerobic step and a dumbbell

Lie on an aerobic step or on the floor, with your knees bent 90 degrees and your feet flat on the floor. Hold a dumbbell with your right hand, arm extended straight up from your body and palm facing in the direction of your feet (1).

Keeping your upper arm stable, slowly bend your right elbow and lower the weight across your chest until the end touches your left shoulder (2). Pause, then straighten your arm and slowly return the weight back to the starting position. Complete one set with your right arm, then switch and repeat with your left.

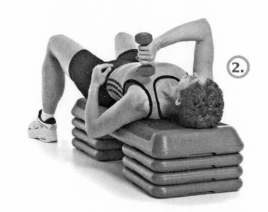

Lift Tips

○ Keep your upper arm and elbow stationary while performing this exercise; do not allow your arm to sway in and out or up and down.

○ Always start with a light weight to get comfortable with the motion and with balancing the weight above you. This will help you avoid stressing your shoulder, an important stabilizer during the exercise.

Shapely Shoulders

The following exercises are designed to strengthen and tone the three deltoid muscles that run along the fronts, tops, and backs of your shoulders. Strong, shapely shoulders are definitely one of the sexiest features of the body. Not to mention that they make everything in life, from typing on a computer to hanging pictures, a whole lot easier.

lateral lift

Rating: BASIC
Equipment: Dumbbells

Stand with your feet hip- to shoulder-width apart. Hold a dumbbell in each hand, allowing your arms to hang down at your sides naturally, with your palms facing in (1).

Keeping your elbows soft, slowly raise your arms out to the sides until they are in line with your shoulders (2). Pause, then lower them back to the starting position.

Lift Tips

○ Lift until the weights are at shoulder level, no higher. Lifting your arms into a V above your head puts too much pressure on your shoulder nerves.

○ Keep a slight bend in your elbows throughout the exercise; don't lock your arms straight out.

○ If you're having trouble keeping your body stable during the exercise, try doing it sitting on the edge of a chair instead of standing.

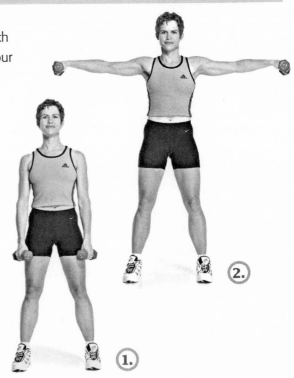

front arm raise

Rating: BASIC
Equipment: Dumbbells

Stand with your feet hip- to shoulder-width apart. Hold a dumbbell in each hand, allowing your arms to hang down at the fronts of your thighs, with your palms facing in (1).

Keeping your elbows slightly bent, slowly raise your right arm in front of you until it is at shoulder height and your palm is facing the floor (2). Pause, then slowly lower it to the starting position. Repeat with your left arm. Alternate arms throughout the exercise, completing an entire set with each arm.

Lift Tips

○ Keep your shoulders down throughout the exercise.

○ Keep your torso stable throughout the exercise. If you find yourself swaying back and forth to lift, the weight is too heavy.

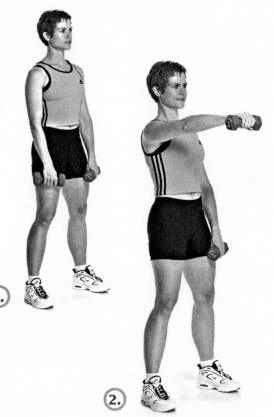

1.

2.

water pitcher fly

Rating: INTERMEDIATE
Equipment: Dumbbells

Stand with your feet hip- to shoulder-width apart. Hold a dumbbell in each hand. With your elbows close to your body, bend your arms straight out in front of you 90 degrees, keeping your palms facing in (1). It should look as though you're holding two water pitchers.

Keeping your hands out in front of you, contract your shoulders and raise your upper arms and elbows out to the side (2). The tops of the weights should rotate toward each other as though you are pouring water out of the pitchers. Pause, then rotate back to the starting position.

Lift Tips

○ Concentrate on keeping your hands straight in line with your forearms throughout the exercise; do not rotate your wrists.

○ Keep your shoulders down while lifting; do not allow them to shrug up toward your ears.

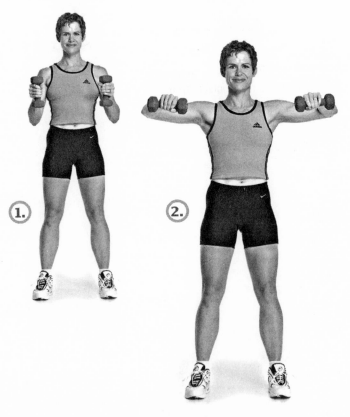

Fabulous Forearms

The following exercises are designed to strengthen and tone the muscles that run down the fronts and backs of your forearms. You use these muscles while performing most exercises, so most people do not make a special attempt to tone them. Sometimes, however, women's forearms are proportionately weaker than their other muscles. If your forearms are the first things to fatigue during an arm curl, tack these exercises onto the end of your routine. Well-toned forearms create beautiful lines from your elbows to your hands.

wrist curl

Rating: BASIC
Equipment: A dumbbell

Sit in a chair with your right hand resting on the side of the chair for support. Hold a weight in your left hand, palm up. Lean your left forearm on your left thigh, with the back of your wrist just slightly over your knee. Let your left wrist bend back naturally with the weight (1).

Using your wrist, curl the weight up and toward your body as far as it will go (2). Pause, then return to the starting position. Complete one set with your left wrist, then switch and repeat with your right.

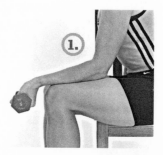

Lift Tips

○ To get more out of this exercise, open your hand slightly as you lower your wrist, so the weight rests across the base of your fingers.

○ This is a small, short motion, so be sure to perform it slowly and deliberately to get the most out of it.

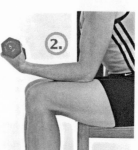

forearm extension

Rating: BASIC
Equipment: A dumbbell

Sit in a chair with your right hand resting under your right knee. Hold a weight in your left hand, palm down. Lean your left forearm on your left thigh with your wrist just slightly over your knee. Let your left wrist bend down toward the floor naturally with the weight (1).

Using your wrist, curl the weight up and toward your body as far as it will go (2). Pause, then return to the starting position. Complete one set with your left wrist, then switch and repeat with your right.

Lift Tips

○ This side of your forearm is typically weaker than the inside, so begin with a light weight.

○ This is a small, short motion, so be sure to perform it slowly and deliberately to get the most out of it.

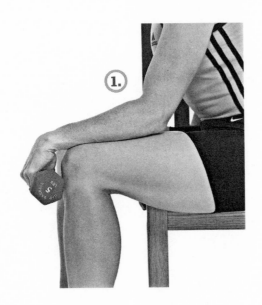 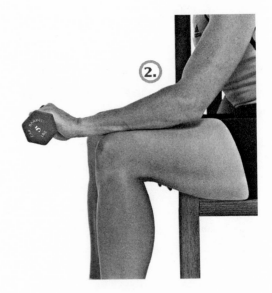

PERFECTLY FIT GOAL:
a tight butt

Making the best of your bottom line

When it comes to firming and toning, the butt can be the final frontier. Many women consider their tushes their biggest trouble zones when it comes to fat loss.

The problem is all the time we spend parked on our rear ends. We once spent our days squatting and standing in the fields, literally working our butts off, but now we sit in front of computer screens, steering wheels, and TVs. And our butts have adapted by giving us bigger, softer cushions to sit on.

What's more, the back end is the female body's fuel pantry. It's where your body stores the fat reserves to draw on when babies need nourishment and food is scarce. Because it serves such an important function, that fat can be stubborn and is often the last to budge.

But don't despair if your back end is a particularly troublesome spot; creating a strong, jiggle-free butt is not impossible. By including a few glute-specific exercises in your training regimen, you can make a visible difference in a short amount of time, especially if you also step up your fat-burning aerobic activity, which helps thin out the fat layer on top of your newly firmed buttocks. And a firm, flab-free butt does more than just sit pretty in your jeans. It gives you the strength to bound up stairs, play tag with your kids, and excel in every sport you play.

Lift, Shape, and Contour

The following exercises are designed to target the gluteal muscles, or the "glutes." These muscles include the gluteus maximus, which makes up the roundest, fullest part of the butt and the lower butt; the gluteus medius, which runs along the outside of the butt and hip area; and the gluteus minimus, which sits between the medius and the maximus. Although these muscles are targeted by the total-body moves discussed in chapter 12, some women feel that they need to give the area "back there" some extra attention.

Getting started. If you're brand new to weight training, incorporate one or two of these exercises into a full-body routine. If you already work out but want a firmer rear, tack on a few of these exercises to your routine. Start with one set of 10 to 12 repetitions and work up to two sets of 12 to 15. Rest for 20 seconds between sets. See "Exercise Ratings" on page 48 to determine which level of exercise is best for you.

What to expect. Expect your butt to burn. Start slowly, and gradually build your reps and sets so that you don't become too sore right from the start.

Safety first. Your back is an important stabilizer during many of these exercises, and you don't want to put too much stress on it. Start with a very light weight or no weight at all until you

between YOU&ME

Start talking booty, and everyone starts shouting about cellulite. As you most likely know, cellulite is basically just fat that bulges between your connective tissues. The best way to shed cellulite is to burn fat and build muscle so that you have fewer bulges and more tone.

You can also try a technique called Endermologie, which uses a vacuumlike machine to gently pull your cellulite-affected tissue into a pair of rolling massager balls. This supposedly stretches the connective fibers, giving your backside a more even appearance. The FDA says the machine can "temporarily reduce the appearance of cellulite." But it's not guaranteed to make your dimples disappear. At 45 minutes and $100 a session, it's a big commitment, especially considering that some doctors say you need about 15 sessions to even start seeing benefits. Buy a pair of running shoes instead.

have the motions down. Perform the exercises slowly, using your muscles, not momentum, to do the work. Keep your back flat and in a neutral position, and avoid any arching or hunching during the exercises.

Results. Perform the exercises 2 or 3 days a week (just not on consecutive days; your muscles need a rest), and you'll feel significantly stronger after just 3 to 6 weeks. After 6 to 8 weeks, you'll start seeing and feeling an improvement in your butt's firmness and appearance.

PERFECTLY FIT TIP

Work your butt while you're parked on it by squeezing your buttocks together as tightly as you can. Hold for 10 to 15 seconds, then relax. Repeat two or three times.

all-fours kickback

Rating: BASIC
Equipment: Ankle weights

Wearing ankle weights, get down on your forearms and knees (similar to the hands-and-knees position, but you bend your arms and support your weight on your forearms instead of your hands). Keep your back straight and your head in line with your back so that your eyes are looking down (1).

Keeping your back straight and leg bent, slowly swing your right leg back and lift your right foot toward the ceiling until your thigh is parallel to the ground (2). Your foot should remain flexed throughout the exercise. Hold for 1 second, then return to the starting position. Do one set with your right leg, then switch and repeat with your left.

Lift Tips

❍ Don't arch or hunch your back during the exercise. This will prevent you from putting stress on your back.

❍ Make the exercise easier by doing it without ankle weights.

❍ Do the exercise with a light dumbbell held behind the knee in the crook of your working leg if you don't have ankle weights.

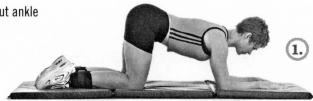

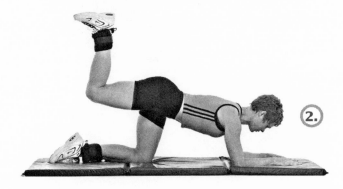

dog walk

Get down on all fours with
your arms fully extended, your palms on the ground, your back straight,
and your head in line with your back so that your eyes are looking
down (1).

Contract your glutes and, keeping your knee bent, raise your left leg
out to the side at a 90-degree angle until it is parallel to the floor (2).
(The position resembles a dog lifting its leg on a fire hydrant, hence the
name Dog Walk.) Pause, then return to the starting position. Do one set
with your left leg, then switch and repeat with your right.

Lift Tips

○ Keep the rest of your body stable while performing the exercise; swaying back
and forth can put unwanted stress on your back.

○ Concentrate on contracting your glutes to perform the movement with maximum effectiveness.

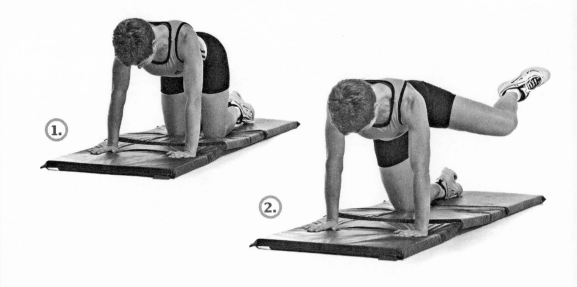

side-lying side kick

Rating: BASIC to INTERMEDIATE
Equipment: None

Lie on your left side, resting your head on your upper arm, and place your right hand on the floor in front of you for support. Bend your lower leg back for balance, and bend your top leg toward your chest, holding it in front of you so that it's parallel to the floor with your foot flexed (1).

Keeping the rest of your body stationary and your top foot flexed, slowly straighten your right leg up and out at a 45-degree angle from your body (2). Pause, then slowly bend the top knee and return your leg to the starting position. Do one set with your right leg, then roll over and repeat with your left.

Lift Tips

○ Avoid swaying forward or back during the exercise; keep your body completely stationary, except for the working leg.

○ Make the exercise more challenging by adding light ankle weights.

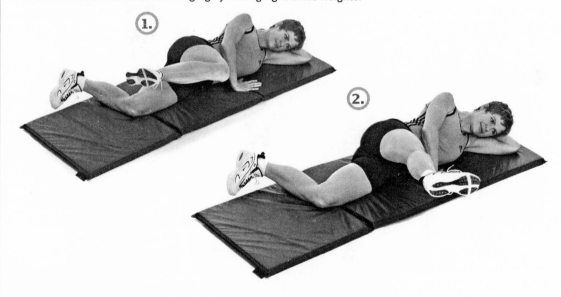

standing press back

Rating: BASIC to INTERMEDIATE
Equipment: Ankle weights and a sturdy chair

Wearing ankle weights, stand facing a sturdy chair with your feet about hip-width apart. Hold on to the chair or table for balance and keep your knees soft (1).

Keeping the rest of your body stable and your hips stationary, contract your glutes and slowly extend your right leg up and back at a 45-degree angle (2). Pause, then slowly return back to the starting position. Do one set with your right leg, then switch and repeat with your left.

Lift Tips

○ Resist the urge to bend way forward while raising your legs. Standing close to your supporting chair can help.

○ Do this exercise by tying an exercise band around your ankles if you don't have ankle weights.

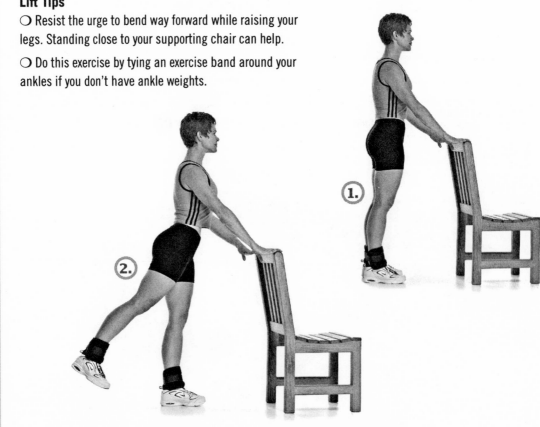

bent-knee crossover

Rating: INTERMEDIATE
Equipment: Ankle weights

Wearing ankle weights, get down on your forearms and knees (similar to the hands-and-knees position, but you bend your arms and support your weight on your forearms instead of your hands). Keep your back straight and your head in line with your back so that your eyes are looking down.

Keeping your knee bent, slowly lift your left leg back until your thigh is parallel to the floor and the sole of your foot is facing the ceiling (1). Then slowly lower your left leg, crossing it over your right calf (2). Pause, then contract your glutes and slowly lift your left thigh back up and lower it to the starting position. Do one set with your left leg, then switch and repeat with your right.

Lift Tips

○ Keep the rest of your body stable while performing the exercise; swaying back and forth can put unwanted stress on your back.

○ Do the exercise with a light dumbbell held behind the knee in the crook of your working leg if you don't have ankle weights.

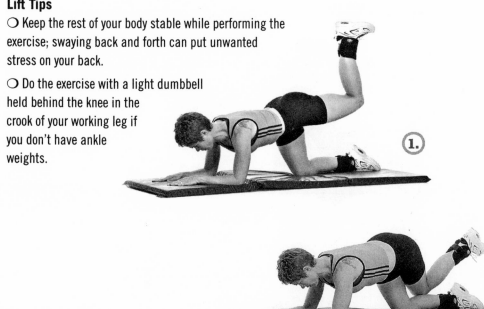

low bridge

Rating: INTERMEDIATE
Equipment: A sturdy chair

Lie on your back on the floor with your legs extended and your heels resting on the edge of a chair seat. Hold your arms straight down by your sides, with your palms down.

Contract your glutes and lift your pelvis up toward the ceiling until your back is in a straight line from your knees to your shoulder blades (1). Raise and straighten your right leg (2). Pause, then lower your leg. Repeat with your left leg on the next lift. Alternate legs until you've done a full set on each side.

Lift Tips

○ Lift only until your back is straight. Don't come up so far that you're up on your neck or that your back is arched. This will keep you from putting stress on your neck or back.

○ Concentrate on contracting your gluteal muscles throughout the entire exercise.

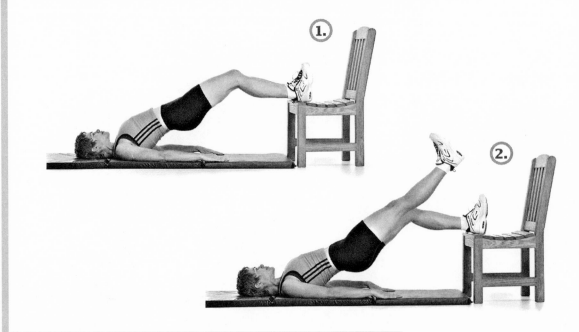

rubber band sidestep

Rating: INTERMEDIATE
Equipment: An exercise band

Stand with your legs about hip-width apart. Loop an exercise band around both ankles (1). It should be tight enough to stay in place, but not so tight that it cuts off your circulation.

Keeping your knees slightly bent and your back straight, take a giant step to the right side with your right foot (2). Then take a small step to the right with your left foot, returning your feet to about hip-width apart, keeping tension on the band. Take a giant step to the left with your left foot, and a small step to the left with your right foot. Keep stepping side to side until you have completed a set on each side.

Lift Tip
○ Keep your head up and eyes facing forward. This will help you avoid the natural tendency to bend forward during this exercise.

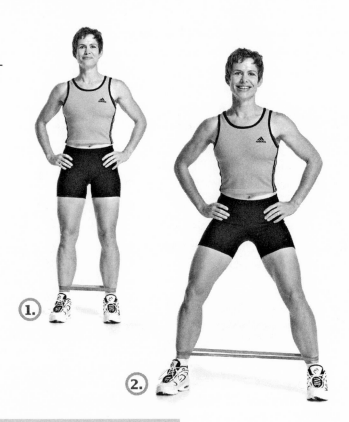

flamingo hip twist

Rating: INTERMEDIATE to ADVANCED
Equipment: A sturdy chair

Stand with your feet about hip-width apart, facing the back of a chair. Lightly hold on to the back of the chair for support and bend your right knee in front of you so that it's almost level with your hips (1).

Slowly swing your knee out to the side, keeping your right foot close to your supporting leg (2). Keeping your right leg bent, lift your right foot back so that your right thigh is out to the side and facing forward (3). Your right thigh and foot should be at hip height, bent at a 45-degree angle with your foot behind you. Hold for 1 second, then slowly return to the starting position. Do one set with your right leg, then switch and repeat with your left.

Lift Tips

❍ Keep your working leg at or just below hip level; this will prevent you from putting excess stress on your back.

❍ Keep your back straight, your head up, and your eyes facing forward, even if you bend forward slightly during the exercise.

❍ Make this exercise more challenging by adding light ankle weights.

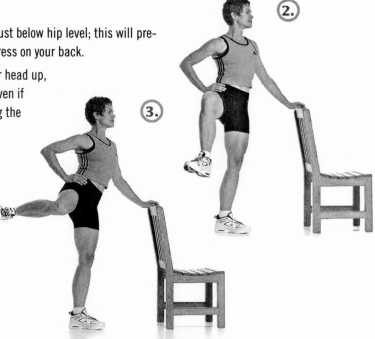

monster walk

Rating: INTERMEDIATE to ADVANCED
Equipment: An exercise band

Stand with your legs hip-width apart. Loop an exercise band around both ankles (1). It should be tight enough to stay in place, but not so tight that it cuts off your circulation.

Bend your knees and take a giant step forward with your left foot (2), immediately followed by a giant step with your right foot. Take 10 giant steps across the room. Pause, then take 10 giant steps backward.

Lift Tips

○ Practice taking giant steps backward first without the band, then with your hand along a table or a wall before you try it unsupported.

○ Bend forward slightly as you do the exercise, to help with balance. Just be sure to keep your back straight, not arched or hunched, as you perform the moves.

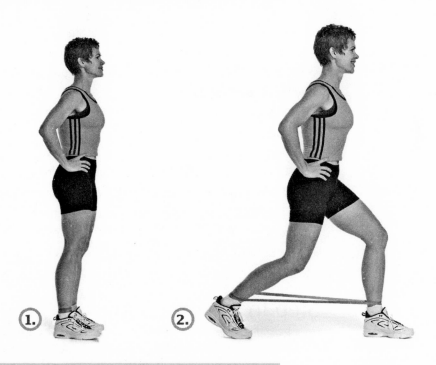

1.   2.

PERFECTLY FIT GOAL:
strong, lean legs
The big payoff

There may be no greater reward for dedicated strength training than strong, toned legs. Solid, shapely thighs and calves put strut in your stride. They let you walk, jump, skate, and climb with ease. They help keep your knees healthy and injury-free. And they look killer in skirts and jeans.

It's no secret that women constantly battle with their legs—especially their thighs. That's because thighs are simply where we are preprogrammed to store fat. And unfortunately, we do a lot of awful things to ourselves trying to make them thin.

The secret to beautiful legs is to stop obsessing about them and start using them the way they were meant to be used. And before you know it, you'll start noticing some firmness here and some sexy curves there.

Does it sound too simple to be true? It's not. It *will* take some energy and dedication. But if you take the time and make the effort, the rewards are fabulous.

Step to a Better Body

Your legs are divided into two sections—your thighs and calves. Your thighs comprise four muscle groups. At the fronts of the thighs are the quadriceps (quads), which

Like many women, I've always wished for impossibly long, Julia Roberts–type legs that just go on forever. All the training in the world won't make you taller, but if you tone your legs, they'll seem longer and leaner.

are the muscles you use to straighten your legs. At the backs are the hamstrings, which you use to bend your legs. The outer-thigh muscles, which include some of your glutes, are the abductors; they pull your legs sideways away from your body. And the adductors, the muscles used to pull your legs sideways back to your body, are in your inner thighs.

You use your quads and hamstrings all the time as you stand, sit, and walk. But unless you participate in activities such as racquetball or skating, your adductors and abductors go largely underused.

The following exercises are designed to work all sides of your legs, strengthening and toning each muscle group to give you fabulously strong legs from every angle.

Getting started. If you're just starting out with weight training, choose two or three of these exercises (include all of the muscles in your legs) to incorporate into a full-body routine. If you already work out but want stronger, more toned calves or thighs, tack on a few of these exercises to your existing routine. Start with one set of 10 to 12 repetitions and work up to two sets of 12 to

15. Rest for 20 seconds between sets. See "Exercise Ratings" on page 48 to determine which level of exercise is best for you.

What to expect. Your quads and hamstrings most likely are stronger than your abductors and adductors. In general, however, women's legs are their strongest body parts and respond well to pushing weight.

Safety first. Knees are the weakest link between strong calf and thigh muscles. This is especially true for women's knees. Keep your knees safe during leg workouts by not allowing them to jut over your toes during squatting motions. Flex and extend your legs in a slow, controlled manner; don't jerk your legs or use momentum to do the work. Since your back is an important stabilizer during lower-body exercise, always keep it flat and in a neutral position, and avoid any arching or hunching during the exercises. The side safety benefit of following these lifting techniques is that your legs will get stronger and ultimately protect your vulnerable knees from injury.

Results. Perform your leg exercises 2 or 3 days a week (just not on consecutive days; your muscles need a rest), and you'll feel significantly stronger after just 3 to 6 weeks. After 6 to 8 weeks, you'll start seeing and feeling an improvement in your legs' firmness and appearance.

PERFECTLY FIT TIP

While sitting at your desk, straighten your right leg, flex your quad, and hold for 10 to 15 seconds. Repeat two or three times, then switch legs.

Sculpted Quads

When toned, the quadriceps form that sexy, sculpted ridge above your knee and up your leg. As a bonus, strong quads help hold your kneecap in line so that you walk, jog, and play injury- and pain-free.

seated straight-leg lift

Rating: BASIC
Equipment: None

Sit on the floor with your right leg extended in front of you, your left leg bent, your back straight, and your feet flexed. Place your hands on the floor behind you for support (1).

Keeping your foot flexed and leg extended, tighten your right quadriceps and slowly raise your right leg up off the floor (2). Pause, then slowly lower your leg back to the floor. Do one set with your right leg, then switch and repeat with your left.

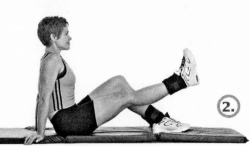

Lift Tips

○ Keep your back flat and in a neutral position; avoid any arching or hunching during the exercise. This will help you avoid stressing your lower back.

○ Concentrate on contracting the quadriceps muscles as hard as you can as you lift and lower.

○ Add light ankle weights to make the exercise more challenging.

leg
extension

Rating: BASIC to INTERMEDIATE
Equipment: Ankle weights and a sturdy chair

Wearing ankle weights, sit on the edge of a chair with your back straight, your legs bent 90 degrees, and your feet flat on the floor. Hold on to the sides of the chair seat for balance and support (1).

Slowly raise and straighten your right leg until it is parallel to the floor and your quadriceps muscles are fully contracted (2). Hold, then slowly lower your leg back to the starting position. Do one set with your right leg, then switch and repeat with your left.

Lift Tips

○ Be careful not to hyperextend your knees and extend your calves past the point where they are parallel to the floor. This is especially important for women, who tend to be more flexible in their joints than men.

○ Use a weight that you can lift and lower in a controlled manner. If you have to kick your leg to get the exercise started, the weight is too heavy.

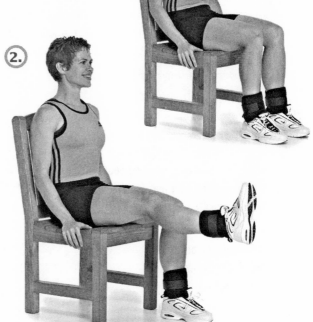

Sexy Hamstrings

When conditioned, the hamstrings form that sexy, sweeping curve down the rear of your legs. As a bonus, you'll walk stronger and ride a bike (even a stationary one) like a pro.

lying leg curl

Rating: BASIC
Equipment: Ankle weights and an optional pillow

Wearing ankle weights, lie face down on the floor. Place a pillow under your hips if that is more comfortable. Rest your head on your forearms for comfort (1).

Slowly bend your right knee and curl your right heel up and in toward your butt (2). Pause, then slowly straighten your leg and lower it back to the starting position. Do one set with your right leg, then switch and repeat with your left.

Lift Tips

○ Concentrate on performing the move slowly and deliberately, using your muscles to lift and lower your leg. Avoid swinging your leg quickly and using momentum to do the work.

○ Keep your foot flexed throughout the exercise for the best results.

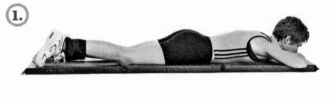

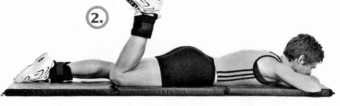

standing hamstring curl

Rating: BASIC to INTERMEDIATE
Equipment: Ankle weights and a sturdy chair

Wearing ankle weights, stand with your feet about hip-width apart, facing the back of a chair. Place your hands on the chair back for support. Keep your back straight, your head aligned with your spine, and your eyes facing forward (1).

Slowly bend your right leg at the knee, raising your heel toward your butt until your shin is parallel to the floor (2). Pause, then lower your leg back to the starting position. Do one set with your right leg, then switch and repeat with your left.

Lift Tips

○ Concentrate on performing the move slowly and deliberately, using your muscles to lift and lower your leg. Avoid swinging your leg quickly and using momentum to do the work.

○ Keep your foot flexed throughout the exercise.

○ Do the exercise with an exercise band tied around your ankles if you don't have ankle weights.

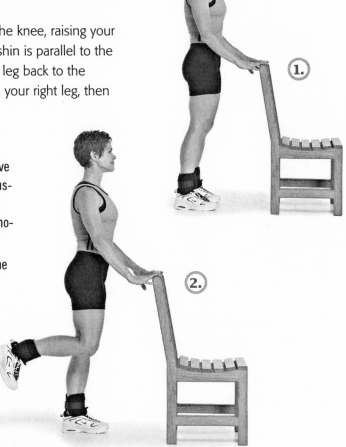

Toned Outer Thighs

The outer thighs are a "problem" area for lots of women. Toning these muscles gives you a sexier silhouette, and as a bonus, you're stronger and more stable during side-to-side activities like tennis and ice skating.

bent-leg raise

Rating: BASIC to INTERMEDIATE
Equipment: Ankle weights

Wearing ankle weights, lie on your left side with your bottom leg straight and your upper leg perpendicular to your body with your knee bent 90 degrees. Both feet should be flexed. Rest your head on your upper arm, and place your right hand on the floor in front of your chest for support (1).

Keeping your top leg bent, raise it up as high as is comfortably possible without twisting your torso or straightening your top leg (2). Pause, then return your leg to the starting position. Do one set with your right leg, then switch and repeat with your left .

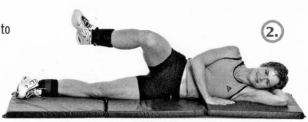

Lift Tips

○ Keep your upper body stationary throughout the exercise; resist the urge to sway back and forth as you lift and lower.

○ Make the exercise easier by doing it without ankle weights first.

v-leg pull

Rating: INTERMEDIATE
Equipment: An exercise band

Loosely tie an exercise band around your ankles and lie on your back with your arms down at your sides. Extend both legs straight up directly above your hips, with your feet spread wide enough that the exercise band is slightly taut (1). Your feet should be flexed.

Slowly open your legs as far as you can (2). When the tension becomes too great to pull any farther, pause, then slowly close your legs back to the starting position.

Lift Tips

○ Keep your back flat on the floor throughout the exercise; do not arch your lower back or twist your torso.

○ Lie next to a chair and hold on to one of its legs for support if balance is a problem.

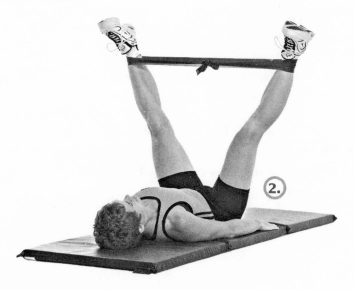

Tight Inner Thighs

The inner thighs are a hot spot for women. When toned, these muscles form strong, lean lines down the insides of your legs. As a bonus, you'll be more stable on your feet.

seated inner-leg lift

Rating: BASIC
Equipment: Ankle weights

Wearing ankle weights, sit on the floor with your hands behind your back for support. Extend your right leg out in front of you and bend your left leg at a 90-degree angle, with your left foot flat on the floor. Rotate your right leg so that your toes point out to the side (1).

Slowly raise your right leg upward as far as comfortably possible (2). Pause, then return your leg to the starting position. Do one set with your right leg, then switch and repeat with your left.

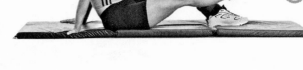

Lift Tips

○ Keep your back straight; avoid any arching or hunching during the exercise.

○ Support your back against a wall instead of with your hands for added comfort.

lying inner-leg lift

Rating: BASIC to INTERMEDIATE
Equipment: Ankle weights

Wearing ankle weights, lie on your left side, resting your head on your upper arm, and place your right hand on the floor in front of your chest for support. Bend the knee of your top leg, placing the foot of that leg in front of your other knee (1). Your bottom leg should be fully extended.

Slowly raise your bottom leg as high as is comfortably possible (2). Hold for 1 second, then slowly lower. Do one set with your left leg, then switch and repeat with your right.

Lift Tips

❍ Keep your upper body stationary throughout the exercise; resist the urge to sway back and forth as you lift and lower.

❍ Do the move without weights to learn the motion, since it can be somewhat awkward at first.

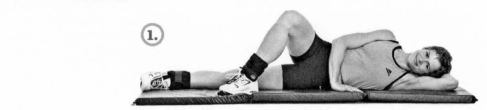

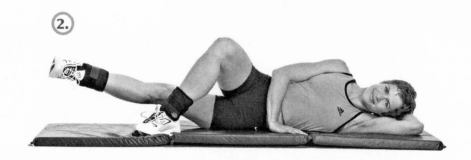

Curvy Calves

The following exercises are designed to strengthen the gastrocnemius and soleus, or calf, muscles as well as the shin muscles in the front of the lower leg. When toned, these muscles give your lower legs a strong, curvy silhouette that looks great in skirts and shorts. As a bonus, you'll have more power in your stride, and you'll be less likely to suffer from shin pain when you walk or run.

If your calves are weak or need toning, simply tack on these exercises to the end of your routine.

calf raise

Rating: BASIC
Equipment: An aerobic step and a dumbbell

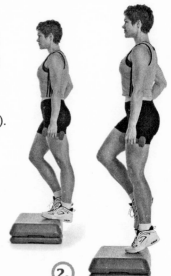

Stand on your left leg with your heel off the edge of a step. You can use the toes of your other leg for balance. Let your left heel drop down as far as it will comfortably go. Hold a dumbbell in your left hand and let it hang naturally by your side (1). If necessary, hold on to a wall or banister with your right hand for support.

Slowly rise up as high as possible on the ball of your left foot (2). Pause, then lower yourself back to the starting position. Do one set with your left foot, then switch and repeat with your right.

Lift Tips

○ Keep your feet pointed forward throughout the exercise to avoid turning your ankles.

○ Use a light weight or no weight at all during the exercise if you can't lift up to your full range of motion.

toe tap

Rating: BASIC
Equipment: A chair

Sit on the edge of a chair with your feet flat on the floor (1). Hold on to the edge of the chair seat for balance and keep your back straight, your head in line with your neck, and your eyes facing forward.

Keeping your heel firmly on the ground, slowly lift your left foot off the floor as far as is comfortably possible (2). Hold, then slowly lower it back to the ground. Do one set with your left foot, then switch and repeat with your right.

Lift Tips

○ Do this exercise three times a week if you tend to get shinsplints during activity.

○ Make this exercise harder by placing the heel of your other foot on top of your working foot and pressing down gently for resistance during the exercise.

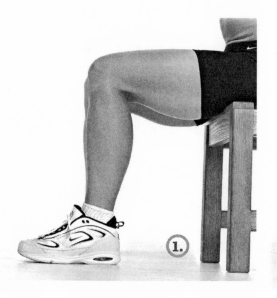

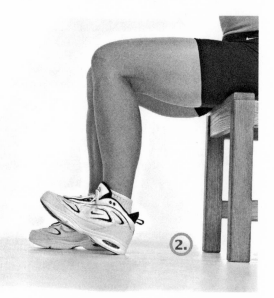

PERFECTLY FIT GOAL:
fab abs

Get a knockout profile

O f all the beautiful muscles in your body, none say, "I kick ass!" more loudly than well-toned abdominals. There are several layers of intricate ab muscles woven together to support your body and hold you upright. When in top shape, these muscles not only cut a stunning profile but they also make you sit and stand straighter and sexier. They support your body so well that you can say "see ya later" to achy back muscles and fatigue. And strong abs look sexy in everything from swimsuits to dress pants.

When you're talking about getting great abs, it's important to make one thing perfectly clear: All the abdominal exercises on the planet will *not* burn off belly fat. These exercises burn calories and build metabolism-boosting muscle, so yes, they'll help. But the real recipe for strong, flat abs is a mixture of daily calorie-burning activity and specific torso-toning exercises. Remember, you can have a rippling showcase of abdominal muscles, but if they're curtained behind a layer of fat, no one will ever see them.

Before menopause, women's abs can remain fairly fat-free, since we tend to stash away extra pounds in our hips and thighs. During and after menopause, however, the hormones responsible for below-the-belt fat storage start to wane, and fat creeps into the abdominal area. You'll shed that tummy bulge with the same exercise no matter what your age—it might just take a little longer if you're postmenopausal.

We've all heard the folks who brag about doing a gazillion situps every day. If you're doing endless abdominal sets and reps, you aren't working your abs hard enough. Instead of increasing your reps and sets, add weight by holding a dumbbell in your hands. Or hold each rep longer in the "up" phase to make your abs work harder.

Twist, Curl, and Tighten

The abdominals are four distinct muscles. First, there's the rectus abdominis, the prominent muscle that runs from just below your chest to your pubic bone. It's separated into eight sections, which create a six-pack effect in lean people when it's toned. It's all one muscle, but there are specific exercises that emphasize both the upper and lower halves of it.

Then there are your internal and external obliques, or the twisting muscles, which run from your ribs to your hips along the front and sides of your torso.

Last are the transverse abdominis, your deepest ab muscles, which run horizontally like tree rings around your torso and help flatten your lower abdominal area.

The following exercises are designed to target one or more of these important abdominal muscles, leaving you with a tight, sculpted midriff.

Getting started. If you're completely new to weight training, choose one to three of these exercises (one for upper abs, one for lower abs, and one for your obliques) to incorporate into a full-body routine. If you already work out but want to target and tighten your abs, tack on a few of these exercises to your existing routine. Start with one set of 10 to 12 repetitions and work up to two sets of 12 to 15. Rest for 20 seconds between sets. See "Exercise Ratings" on page 48 to determine which level of exercise is best for you.

What to expect. The first few repetitions in a set of abdominal exercises are usually pretty easy, but they should become more difficult as you approach the end of your set. Think of your abs as the engine of the exercise. Contract them a bit to start; then further contract them to pull your shoulders and head off the floor.

Safety first. Correct form is essential for ab exercises to both work and be safe. Don't pull on your neck during the exercises, and keep your chin about a fist's distance from your chest. Keep your movements slow and controlled; avoid jerking your body around or using momentum to do the work. Keep your back pressed flat against the floor throughout the exercises.

Results. Perform your abdominal exercises 2 or 3 days a week (just not on consecutive days; your muscles need a rest), and you'll feel significantly tighter and stronger after just 2 to 3 weeks. After 4 to 6 weeks, you should start seeing marked improvements, provided you aren't carrying excess weight in your abdominal area.

PERFECTLY FIT TIP

Keep your ab muscles lightly contracted all day long to maintain good posture and create a strong, lean profile.

Rippling Rectus Abdominis

Some of these exercises focus on either the upper or lower portion of the rectus abdominis; some target both parts. If you work the entire region, you'll have a rippling washboard when it's toned. As a bonus, you won't need a hand getting up off the floor anymore.

2-second floor crunch

Muscles worked: Upper abs
Rating: BASIC
Equipment: None

Lie on your back with your feet resting flat on the floor, your knees bent at a 90-degree angle, your hands clasped lightly behind your head, and your elbows out to the sides. Tilt your pelvis slightly to flatten your back against the floor (1).

Contract your abs and slowly lift your shoulders and head off the floor about 30 degrees (2). Hold for 2 seconds, then lower them back to the starting position.

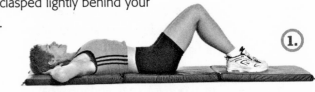
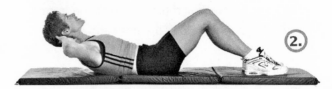

Lift Tips

❍ Do not pull on your neck during the exercise. To avoid neck strain, keep your chin forward (you should always be able to fit a fist between your chin and your chest) and your eyes facing the ceiling.

❍ Raise yourself off the floor very slowly, pause for 2 seconds at the top, then lower yourself very slowly. This will give you the best results.

chair curl

Muscles worked: Upper abs
Rating: BASIC
Equipment: A sturdy chair

Lie on your back with your feet up on a chair so that your knees are bent at a 90-degree angle. Place your hands behind your head and hold your elbows out to the sides (1).

Press your heels down onto the chair and contract your abs to raise your ribs, chest, and shoulders off the floor about 30 degrees (2). Hold, then lower yourself back to the starting position.

Lift Tips

○ Do not pull on your neck during this exercise. To avoid neck strain, keep your chin forward (you should always be able to fit a fist between your chin and your chest) and your eyes facing the ceiling.

○ Raise yourself off the floor very slowly, pause for 2 seconds at the top, then lower yourself very slowly. This will give you the best results.

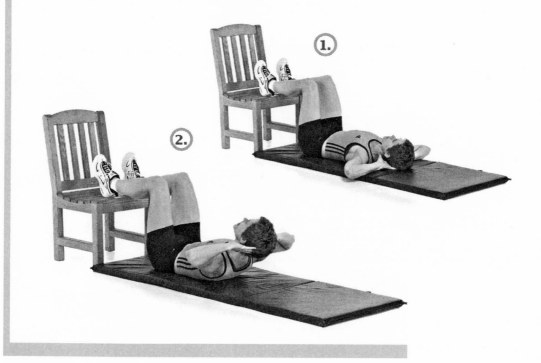

reverse curl

Muscles worked: Lower abs
Rating: BASIC to INTERMEDIATE
Equipment: None

Lie flat on your back with your hands clasped lightly behind your head and your elbows out to the sides. Raise your legs so that your thighs are perpendicular to your body and your calves are parallel to the floor. Tilt your pelvis slightly to flatten your back against the floor.

In a slow, controlled manner, raise your hips toward your rib cage so that your knees drop toward your forehead. Hold, then slowly lower yourself back to the starting position.

Lift Tips

○ Keep your abs contracted throughout the exercise.

○ Concentrate on curling your pelvic bone toward your rib cage; do not just lower and raise your legs. This will help you get the most out of the exercise.

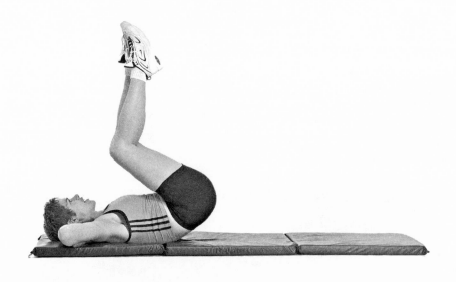

in and out

Muscles worked: Upper and lower abs
Rating: INTERMEDIATE
Equipment: None

Lie on your back with your feet resting flat on the floor and your knees bent at a 90-degree angle. Clasp your hands lightly behind your head with your elbows out to the sides. Tilt your pelvis slightly to flatten your back against the floor.

Contract your upper and lower abs and slowly raise your hips toward your rib cage so that your knees come up toward your chest. At the same time, raise your shoulders and head off the floor (1). Hold for 1 second. Keeping your legs raised, slowly lower your shoulders back to the floor while dropping your hips and slightly extending your legs (2). Hold, then curl again. Repeat this in-and-out motion throughout the set.

Lift Tips

○ Concentrate on curling in and opening your body back down and out in one fluid motion.

○ Keep your head back and avoid tucking your chin into your chest during the exercise.

○ Don't extend your legs as far if your lower back aches during this move.

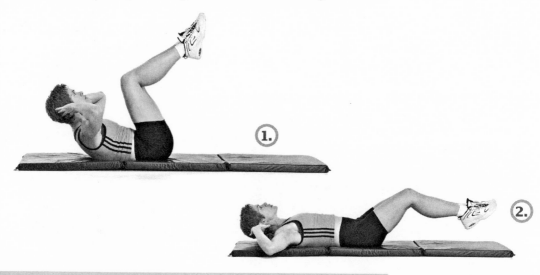

hand-to-foot ball curl

Muscles worked: Upper and lower abs
Rating: ADVANCED
Equipment: A large, light ball like an inflated exercise ball, basketball, or soccer ball

Lie on the floor with your legs straight in front of you and your knees slightly bent. Hold an exercise ball (or another light, large ball like a basketball) in both hands and extend your arms back over your head (1).

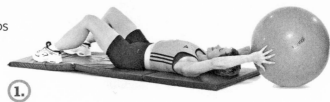

1.

Contract your upper and lower abs and raise your arms and legs toward one another, straightening your legs as you do but keeping your knees soft. When your hands and feet are directly over your body, move the ball from your hands to your feet (2), then simultaneously and slowly lower your arms and legs back to the starting position (3). Repeat, this time switching the ball from your feet to your hands at the "up" position.

Lift Tips

◯ Spend some time doing basic and intermediate exercises to build strength in your upper and lower rectus abdominis if you feel stress on your lower back.

◯ Keep your head back and avoid tucking your chin into your chest during the exercise.

◯ Raise and lower your arms and legs as simultaneously as possible for the best results.

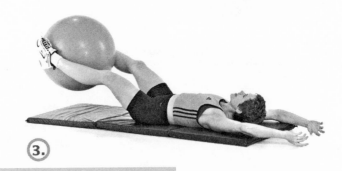

2.

3.

partner ball toss

Muscles worked: Upper and lower abs
Rating: ADVANCED
Equipment: A medicine ball

Lie on your back with your feet resting flat on the floor and your knees bent at a 90-degree angle. Hold a medicine ball in both hands just above your chest. Tilt your pelvis slightly to flatten your back against the floor. Have your partner stand at your feet, facing you.

All in one motion, contract your abdominals and slowly lift your shoulders and head off the floor about 30 degrees, extend your arms, and toss the ball to your partner. Pause in the "up" position with your arms still outstretched. Have your partner toss the ball back to you, then slowly bring the ball back to your chest as you lower yourself to the floor.

Lift Tips

❍ Soften your elbows to absorb some of the impact when catching the ball.

❍ Keep your head back and avoid tucking your chin into your chest during the exercise.

❍ Raise, throw, catch, and lower in fluid, smooth moves.

❍ Make the exercise harder by starting with the ball extended back over your head, raising it up and over your head to toss it, and bringing it up and back with you to lower it.

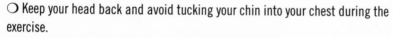

Oh, What Obliques

Well–toned obliques give your torso strong, curvy lines. As a bonus, you'll throw a punch meaner than Ms. Ali!

alternating twisting crunch

Rating: INTERMEDIATE
Equipment: None

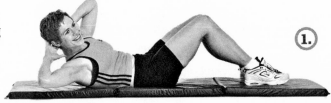

Lie on your back with your feet resting flat on the floor, your knees bent at a 90-degree angle, your hands clasped lightly behind your head, and your elbows out to the sides. Tilt your pelvis slightly to flatten your back against the floor.

Slowly bring your left shoulder off the ground as you cross your left elbow in the direction of your right knee (1). Hold, then slowly return to the starting position. Repeat the motion going from right to left (2). Alternate sides throughout the exercise until you have done a full set on each side.

Lift Tips

❍ Do not pull on your neck during this exercise. To avoid neck strain, keep your chin forward (you should always be able to fit a fist between your chin and your chest), your elbows out wide, and your eyes facing the ceiling.

❍ Keep the motion slow; do not jerk your body back and forth.

torso twist

Rating: INTERMEDIATE to ADVANCED
Equipment: A medicine ball

Lie on your back with your legs bent so that your thighs are perpendicular and your calves are parallel to the floor at a 90-degree angle. Squeeze a medicine ball between your knees and hold your hands behind your head, with your elbows out to the sides (1).

Slowly lower your knees to the right about 45 degrees, or until you feel a stretch (2). Hold for a few seconds, then raise them back to the starting position. Alternate sides throughout the exercise until you have done a full set on each side.

Lift Tips

○ Make the exercise more difficult by maintaining a crunch position with your shoulders and head 30 degrees off the floor throughout the exercise.

○ Do the exercise with a regular basketball or volleyball if you don't have a medicine ball or the medicine ball is too heavy.

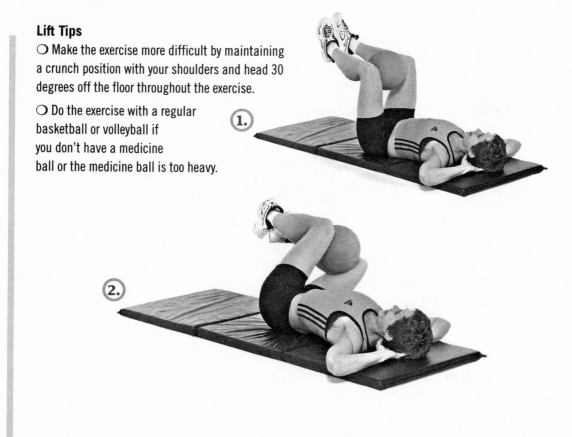

Sculpted Front and Sides

The following exercises are designed to give you more bang for your buck by hitting most of the abdominal muscles at once. They're a little tough for beginners, but if you have fairly strong abdominal muscles, these can offer a great new challenge.

floor side bend

Rating: BASIC TO INTERMEDIATE
Equipment: A sturdy chair

Lie on your back with your feet up on a chair so that your knees are bent at a 90-degree angle. Place your hands behind your head and hold your elbows out to the sides.

Press your heels down onto the chair. Slowly raise your upper back, shoulders, and head off the floor about 30 degrees. Hold, then bend sideways at the waist to the left. Come back to center, then slowly bend sideways to the right. Lower yourself back to the starting position.

Lift Tips

❍ Do not pull on your neck during the exercise. To avoid neck strain, keep your chin forward (you should always be able to fit a fist between your chin and your chest) and your eyes facing the ceiling.

❍ Keep your lower back flat against the floor throughout the entire exercise.

circle crunch

Rating: ADVANCED
Equipment: A medicine ball

Lie on your back with your legs bent so that your thighs are perpendicular and your calves are parallel to the floor at a 90-degree angle. Squeeze a medicine ball between your knees and hold your hands behind your head, with your elbows out to the sides (1).

Contract your abs and raise your upper back, shoulders, and head off the floor about 30 degrees. Slowly move your knees in a counterclockwise circular motion (2). Repeat for a half-set (about 5 circles). Pause, then slowly move your knees in a clockwise circular motion.

Lift Tips

○ Keep your back flat on the floor throughout the entire exercise.

○ Do the exercise with a regular basketball or volleyball if you don't have a medicine ball or the medicine ball is too heavy.

○ Make the exercise more difficult by making wider circles with your knees.

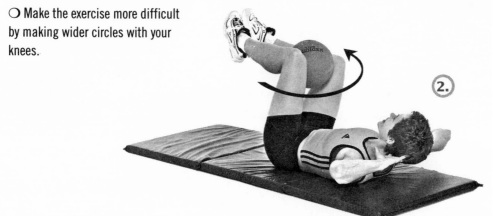

PERFECTLY FIT GOAL:
a strong, bareable back

Suddenly slimmer

f someone asked you to name the body part you would most like to tone and strengthen, chances are you'd never say, "My back." But every woman's back is brimming with beautiful muscles just waiting to be developed. These muscles not only give you a sensational rear view but they also make you stand taller, play sports better, ache less, and appear leaner. Because there's relatively little fat back there, and because those muscles tend to be fairly weak from underuse, you can get visible results in just a few weeks.

And before you ask: No, you won't get bulky. Instead, you'll trade in a wimpy upper body that makes your hips and thighs look disproportionately big for a toned, curvy torso that'll instantly make your hips and thighs look trimmer. You'll also slump less and feel stronger even when you're just sitting at your desk.

To tone your back correctly, you need exercises that work it from every angle. Your back is made up of an interwoven system of four muscles that help you lift, pull, sit, and stand up straight. The biggest and most visible is the latissimus dorsi, or the lats, a fan-shaped muscle that runs from your lower spine under your arms to the fronts of your shoulders. When well-toned, the lats give your torso a strong, athletic V-shape.

Next to the lats is the trapezius, or traps, which runs from the mid- and upper spine up and out to your neck and shoulders.

Supporting the traps are your rhomboids, which extend from your upper spine to your shoulders and help to hold your chest open and prevent your shoulders from hunching forward.

Completing the picture are your erector spinae, or erectors. These muscles run the length of your spine from your tailbone to your upper back, giving you good standing posture and keeping your lower back strong and pain-free when they're conditioned.

Building a Balanced Body

The following exercises are specifically designed to home in on all four areas of your back: lats, traps, rhomboids, and erectors. As you integrate these exercises into your strength-training routine, you'll develop a more balanced body.

Getting started. If you're brand new to weight training, choose two or three of these exercises (making sure all four muscle groups are worked) to incorporate into a full-body routine. If you already work out but want a sexier back or better posture, tack on a few of these exercises to your existing routine. Start with one set of 10 to 12 repetitions and work up to two sets of 12 to 15. Rest for 20 seconds between sets. See "Exercise Ratings" on page 48 to determine which level of exercise is best for you.

PERFECTLY FIT TIP

When you feel hunched over, squeeze your shoulder blades together and contract your upper-back muscles. Hold for 10 to 15 seconds, then relax.

What to expect. Some back exercises will be a piece of cake, while others leave you limp. That's because we tend to have a lot of muscular imbalance back there. Just adjust your weights accordingly. Also, it's very easy to "cheat" during back workouts without even knowing it. Many exercises use your back muscles to "row" weights toward your body. Although it's tempting to use your arms to assist, that won't help your back. Always concentrate on initiating the moves with your back muscles, contracting them first and letting your arms help out at the end.

Safety first. These exercises will help give you a strong, healthy back, but it's important to do them correctly and with proper form. Always keep your back straight and your head and neck in line with your spine. Don't arch or round your lower back or hunch your shoulders. Your torso should be stable as you lift and lower the weights, so avoid jerking your body or using momentum to do the work. Always begin with light weights to get comfortable with the exercises.

Results. Perform your back exercises 2 or 3 days a week (just not on consecutive days; your muscles need a rest), and you'll feel stronger in just 2 to 4 weeks. After 4 to 6 weeks, you'll start seeing results.

lat pulldown

Muscles worked: Latissimus dorsi and rhomboids
Rating: BASIC
Equipment: An exercise band

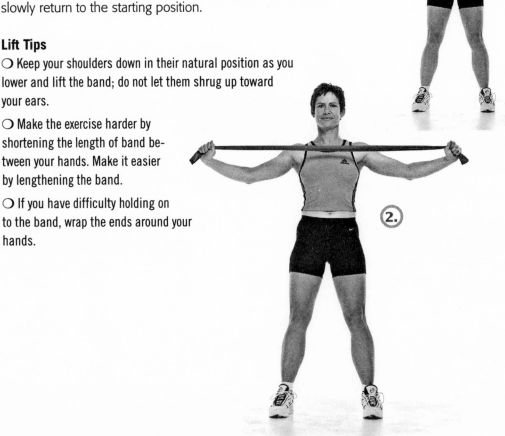

1.

2.

Stand with your feet slightly wider than shoulder-width apart. Hold the ends of an exercise band (if you don't have a long exercise band, tie two together) and hold the band over your head with your hands outstretched (1).

Keeping your arms straight, but elbows slightly soft, pull and lower the band down in front of your face—being careful not to let the band hit you in the face—until your arms are completely outstretched and the band is at chest level (2). Pause, then slowly return to the starting position.

Lift Tips

○ Keep your shoulders down in their natural position as you lower and lift the band; do not let them shrug up toward your ears.

○ Make the exercise harder by shortening the length of band between your hands. Make it easier by lengthening the band.

○ If you have difficulty holding on to the band, wrap the ends around your hands.

weighted shrug

Muscles worked: Trapezius
Rating: BASIC
Equipment: Dumbbells

Stand with your feet shoulder-width apart with your back straight and your knees soft for support. Hold a dumbbell in each hand, allowing your arms to hang down naturally at your sides, with your palms facing in toward your thighs (1).

Slowly shrug your shoulders straight up toward your ears (2). Pause, then lower them back to the starting position.

Lift Tips

❍ Avoid putting excess stress on your shoulder joints by being careful to lift your shoulders up and down in a vertical line; do not rotate them forward or backward.

❍ Use a weight that is heavy enough that your traps get fatigued by the end of your set, but not so heavy that you can't raise your shoulders up to their full range of motion.

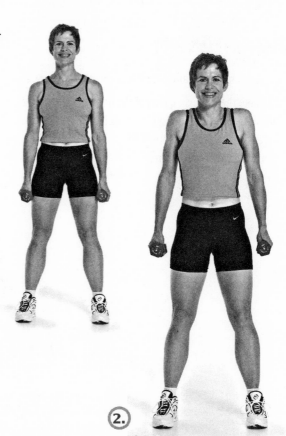

1.

2.

across-the-chest pull

Muscles worked: Latissimus dorsi and rhomboids
Rating: BASIC
Equipment: An exercise band

Stand with your feet shoulder-width apart, with your back straight and your knees soft. Wrap the ends of an exercise band around each hand and hold your arms straight out from your body in front of you, with your hands slightly wider than shoulder-width apart and your elbows slightly bent (1).

Slowly squeeze your shoulder blades together and pull the exercise band across your chest until your arms are out to your sides (2). Pause, then slowly return to the starting position.

Lift Tips

○ Keep the band taut throughout the entire exercise.

○ Make the exercise more challenging by shortening the length of band. Always start with your hands wider than shoulder-width apart to avoid putting stress on your shoulders.

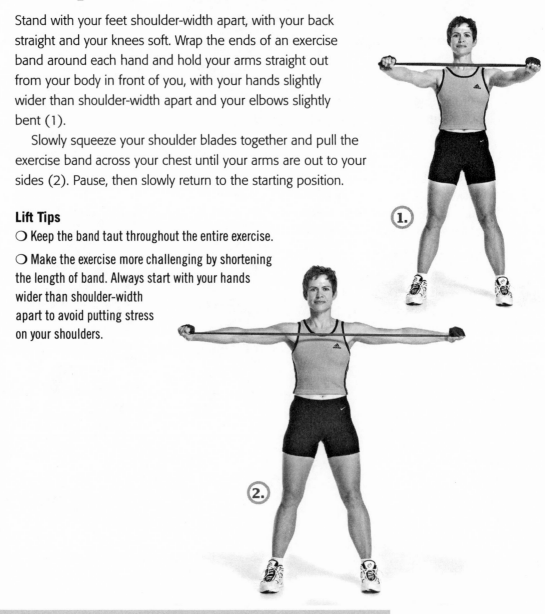

superwoman

Muscles worked: Erector spinae
Rating: INTERMEDIATE
Equipment: None

Lie facedown with your legs extended straight behind you, your toes pointed, and your arms extended straight over your head. Hold your head straight in line with your spine, and keep your chin up off the floor at a comfortable level.

Slowly raise your right arm and your left leg at the same time until they are both a few inches off the floor. Hold, then slowly lower them back to the starting position. Repeat with the opposite arm and leg. Alternate arms and legs throughout the exercise until you have done a half-set (about 10 reps) to each side.

Lift Tips

○ Be careful not to strain your lower-back muscles by lifting your arms and legs higher than is comfortably possible.

○ Make the exercise more difficult by using light dumbbells and ankle weights.

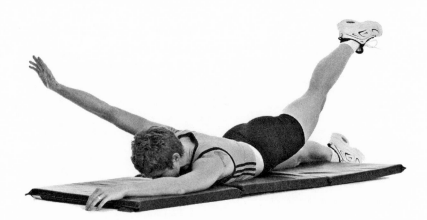

reverse grip row

Muscles worked: Latissimus dorsi, trapezius, and rhomboids
Rating: ADVANCED
Equipment: A sturdy chair and a dumbbell

Stand facing the back of a sturdy chair with a dumbbell in your right hand and your left hand holding onto the chair back for support. Bend your knees slightly and bend forward from the waist at a 45-degree angle. Hold the dumbbell out in front of you with your palm up and your hand positioned lower than your left hand (1).

Slowly pull the dumbbell up toward your body until it touches your hip bone (2). Pause, then slowly lower it back to the starting position. Do one set with your right hand, then switch and repeat with your left.

Lift Tips

○ If you have lower-back troubles, skip the exercise since it relies heavily on your lower back for support.

○ Keep your back flat, your head in line with your spine, and your eyes facing forward throughout the exercise.

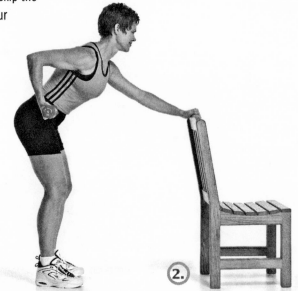

reverse extension

Muscles worked: Erector spinae
Rating: ADVANCED
Equipment: An aerobic step or bench

Lie facedown on an aerobic step or bench, allowing your legs to hang down off the edge with your hips bent at a 45- to 90- degree angle. Bend your knees and cross your ankles. Hold on to the edges of the step for support. Keep your head down and in line with your spine (1).

Keeping your knees bent, slowly lift your legs until your thighs are in line with your body and are parallel to the floor (2). Pause, then slowly lower them back to the starting position.

Lift Tips

○ Avoid lower back strain by keeping your movements slow and controlled; do not jerk your legs up and down.

○ Help support your lower back during the exercise by keeping your abdominals tight throughout the movement.

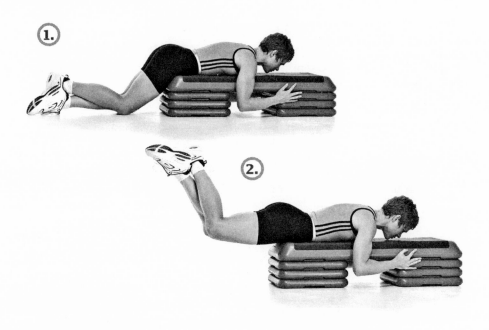

PERFECTLY FIT GOAL:
killer cleavage

Keeping your chest high and mighty

f you're a woman, you have worried about your chest. In a culture that uses gigantic boobs to sell everything from bubble gum to BMWs, it's practically impossible not to. What really stinks, though, is that by the time most women learn to accept the size of their breasts, they've reached the age where they start worrying about succumbing to the effects of gravity, aging, and pregnancy.

As one client put it, "If I can just keep them up where they belong, I'll be happy!"

The good news is that strength training can help. No, it can't change the breast tissue itself because that's fat. And since you can't shape fat, the structure of your breasts will remain largely the same. But what you can do is build up the muscles that lie behind your breasts. This not only will fill out your chest area and give your bustline a lift but also it will create an illusion of cleavage, even if you're not naturally endowed.

What's more, strong pectoral muscles, or pecs, do more than just look nice. A strong chest gives you the power to push heavy shopping carts, throw a wicked left hook, and give your mate a serious squeeze.

Working the Angles

Your chest is made up of three muscles—the pectoralis major, the pectoralis minor, and the serratus anterior. They're all important, but for a sexier and stronger chest, the muscle to target is the pectoralis major. This muscle blankets most of your chest area, fanning out from your shoulders and spreading to your collarbone, your breastbone, and your ribs. Because it's so big, it's difficult to challenge the entire muscle with one exercise. For the best results, target the upper pecs, the area above your breasts, with some exercises, and the center pecs, the area right beneath your breasts, with others.

The following exercises are designed to target your pectoral muscles from different angles to give you the dual benefit of elongated cleavage, from both nicely defined upper pecs and the full-breasted appearance of well-developed center pecs.

Getting started. If you're brand new to weight training, choose one or two of these exercises to target either your upper pecs or your center pecs, depending on your goals, to incorporate into a full-body routine. If you already work out but want a stronger, fuller chest, tack on a few of these exercises to your existing routine. Start with one set of 10 to 12 repetitions and work up to two sets of 12 to 15 reps. Rest for 20 seconds between sets. See "Exercise Ratings" on page 48 to determine which level of exercise is best for you.

What to expect. Most of these exercises are fairly straightforward and can be mastered with ease. The presses and flies might be a little tricky

PERFECTLY FIT TIP

Give your chest a boost with wall pushups. Stand about 2 feet from a wall and lean against it with your back straight and palms at the sides of your chest against the wall. Do a set of 15 pushups. Relax, then repeat.

for new lifters only because they require a little bit of coordination to balance the weights while lifting and lowering them. But after a few sessions, that slightly wobbly feeling will disappear.

Safety first. Chest exercises also challenge the shoulders, so it's important to take some precautions not to overstress your more delicate rotator cuff (supporting shoulder) muscles. As you press the weights in a chest press or close your arms in a fly, concentrate on squeezing your chest muscles so that you use those muscle fibers, not your arms and shoulders, to do the work. Keep your shoulders down and back as much as possible to lessen their involvement. Maintain a slight bend in your elbows, especially during flies, to prevent joint strain. Lower the weights only to just above chest level, not lower. Finally, keep your back straight and flat while lifting. If you have to arch your back to lift the weights, they're too heavy.

Results. The chest responds quickly to strength training. Perform your pec exercises 2 or 3 days a week (just not on consecutive days; your muscles need a rest), and you'll feel stronger in just 2 to 3 weeks. After 3 to 4 weeks, you'll start seeing results.

dumbbell side swing

Muscles worked: Center pecs
Rating: BASIC
Equipment: A dumbbell

Stand with your feet shoulder-width apart, with your knees slightly bent for support. Hold a dumbbell in your right hand and raise your arm out to the side at shoulder level, with your palm facing down. Hold your left hand on your hip for support (1).

Keeping your elbow slightly bent, slowly contract your chest muscles and bring your arm around so that the weight ends up straight out in front of your body (2). Pause, then slowly return your arm to the starting position. Do one set with your right arm, then switch and repeat with your left.

Lift Tips

○ Use a light weight, since this exercise relies heavily on your shoulder muscles and connective tissues.

○ Concentrate on squeezing your chest muscles to slowly move your arm to and fro; let your shoulders do the supporting work.

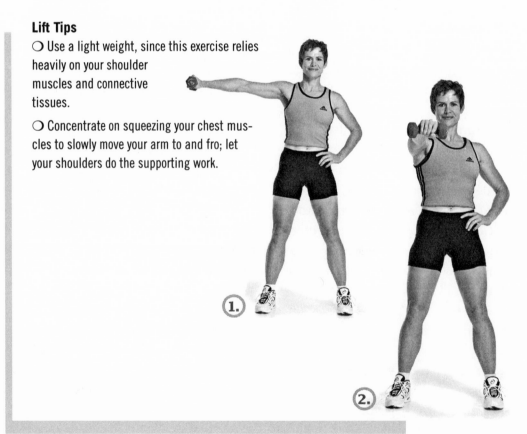

chest fly

Muscles worked: Center pecs
Rating: BASIC
Equipment: An optional aerobic step or bench and dumbbells

Lie on your back on an aerobic step or bench (the floor is fine if neither is available, but the exercise will be less effective) with your feet flat on the floor. Hold a pair of dumbbells up over your chest with your arms extended and your palms facing in toward each other. Keep your elbows slightly bent.

Slowly open your arms out to the sides, allowing the weights to fall to about the 9 o'clock and 3 o'clock positions. Pause, then slowly close your arms back to the starting position. Keep your shoulders down and back throughout the move.

Lift Tips

❍ Do not let the weights drop below chest level; doing so puts too much stress on your shoulders.

❍ Use a lighter weight for a fly than you would for a press because the fly uses fewer muscles to do the work.

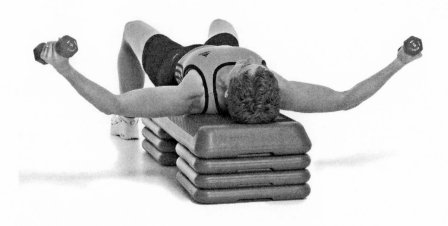

single-arm crossover

Muscles worked: Center and upper pecs
Rating: BASIC to INTERMEDIATE
Equipment: An exercise band and a sturdy door

Tie an exercise band around the knob of a sturdy door. Stand far enough away from the door so that the band is taut. Turn so that your left side is facing the door, and loop the end of the exercise band around your left hand. Position your feet about shoulder-width apart, keep your back straight, and bend slightly from the waist (1). Your left arm should be slightly bent and out about 45 degrees from your side.

Slowly contract your chest muscles and keeping your elbow slightly bent, pull the band across your body in a semicircular motion (2). Hold, then slowly return to the starting position. Do one set with your left arm, then switch and repeat with your right.

Lift Tips

❍ Keep your back straight and in a neutral position; avoid any arching or hunching during the exercises.

❍ Make the exercise more challenging by shortening the amount of band between you and the door. Make it easier by lengthening the band.

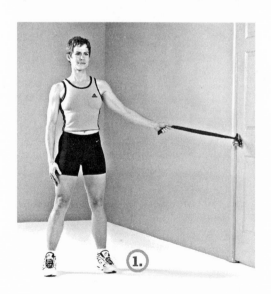

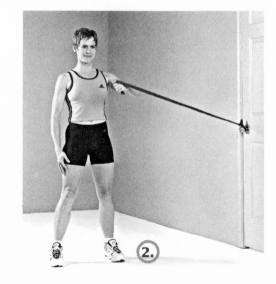

incline press

Muscles worked: Upper pecs	

Muscles worked: Upper pecs
Rating: INTERMEDIATE
Equipment: Dumbbells and an aerobic step, a bench, or a large, inflated exercise ball

The goal here is to support your body in an incline position. An adjustable lifting bench is the best solution. If you don't have access to one, either stack up one side of an aerobic step and push it against the wall for support or position yourself on an exercise ball so that your shoulders and upper back are on the top of the ball and the rest of your body is on an incline with your hips positioned lower. Keep your legs bent and your feet flat on the floor. Once you're in an incline position, hold the dumbbells straight up over your chest with your arms extended, your palms facing the ceiling and your thumbs facing each other.

Slowly lower the weights so that your elbows point down and out perpendicular to your body. Stop when the weights are about even with your chest. Slowly return to the starting position, bringing the weights together as you do. Pause, then lower them again.

Lift Tips

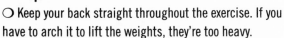

❍ Keep your back straight throughout the exercise. If you have to arch it to lift the weights, they're too heavy.

❍ Use light weights the first few times to get the hang of the motion if you feel a little shaky the first time you try the exercise.

❍ Use an exercise band for this exercise if you don't have a step, a bench, or a ball. Simply loop the band around your back.

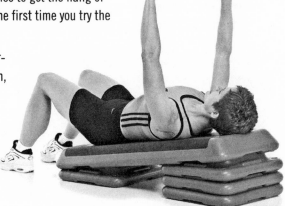

incline fly

Muscles worked: Upper pecs
Rating: INTERMEDIATE
Equipment: Dumbbells and an aerobic step, a bench, or a large, inflated exercise ball

This exercise requires that you support your body in an incline position. An adjustable lifting bench is the best solution. If you don't have access to one, either stack up one side of an aerobic step and push it against the wall for support or position yourself on an exercise ball so that your shoulders and upper back are on the top of the ball and the rest of your body is on an incline with your hips positioned lower. Keep your legs bent and your feet flat on the floor. Once you're in an incline position, hold the dumbbells up over the upper portion of your chest with your arms extended and your palms facing in toward each other. Keep your elbows slightly bent.

Slowly open your arms out to the sides, allowing the weights to fall to the 9 o'clock and 3 o'clock positions. Pause, then slowly close your arms back to the starting position. Keep your shoulders down and back throughout the move.

Lift Tips

○ Use a lighter weight for a fly than you would for a press because the fly uses fewer muscles to do the work.

○ Concentrate on squeezing your chest muscles and using them, not your shoulders, to lift and lower the weights.

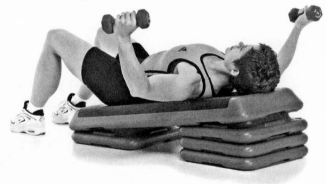

alternating one-arm chest press

Muscles worked: Center pecs
Rating: ADVANCED
Equipment: An optional aerobic step or bench and dumbbells

Lie on your back on an aerobic step or bench (the floor is fine if neither is available, but the exercise will be less effective) with your feet flat on the floor. With your right hand, hold a dumbbell up over your chest with your arm extended and your palm facing the ceiling so that the dumbbell is positioned horizontally. With your left hand, hold a dumbbell down at the left side of your chest so that the weight is positioned vertically.

Slowly lower the right weight, rotating your wrist as you come toward your body, so that the weight ends up positioned vertically at the side of your chest. Immediately press the left weight up, rotating your wrist so that your arm ends up extended with the dumbbell positioned horizontally. Pause, then lower the left weight back to the starting position. Continue alternating until you have done a full set to each side.

Lift Tips

❍ Begin with light weights, since the exercise requires a fair amount of joint stability and balance.

❍ Keep your back flat throughout the exercise. If you have to hike your hips or arch your back, the weight is too heavy.

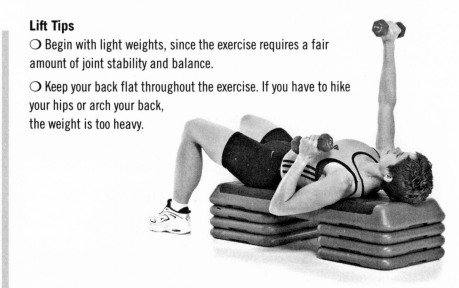

essential stretches

Limber muscles, calm mind in just 10 minutes a day

Anyone who says she doesn't skimp on stretching is either in love with her yoga class or she's lying. I don't mean to put anyone down; it's just that stretching is the one key element to fitness that people forget about. In fact, the American Council on Exercise named "neglecting to stretch" the mistake folks make most often while getting in shape.

I promise that you have time to work out *and* stretch. It takes no more than 10 minutes a day, and the payoffs are enormous.

The Many Benefits of a Limber Body

Stretching will make you feel better, especially if you're working out and weight training. Muscles remember the last thing you do. And if the last thing you've done is contract them over and over while running, bicycling, or pressing dumbbells, they'll end up tighter and shorter.

What's more, every muscle in your body contains "stretch receptors" that keep a constant dialogue going with your brain about your overall level of tension. When your muscles are chronically tight, your body is thrown out of alignment, creating muscular imbalances and poor posture. That notifies your brain that your body is under constant stress. Can you say tension headache?

Stretching also makes your body perform better. You'll gain a greater range of motion, so you can generate more force. Your stride will be longer, your golf swing will be stronger, and you'll think nothing of taking the stairs two at a time. Even everyday stuff like tying your shoes will be easier. But more important, flexible muscles also help prevent muscle soreness and injury.

Aesthetically, well-stretched and limber muscles appear leaner than shortened, constantly contracted muscles. Stretching also undoes a lot of the postural damage we do even when we're not working out.

Finally, stretching has some hidden psychological benefits. Just as chronically tight muscles send a signal to your brain that you're under constant stress, "chronically" relaxed muscles send the opposite message, telling your brain that everything is okay. That can make you feel less stressed out even when things are crazy. Plus, when done properly, stretching simply feels good.

How to Get a Good Stretch

Stretching is as simple to do as bending and breathing. Before you begin, here are six rules of thumb to keep in mind as you reach for a longer, more limber body.

1. Stretch warm. As eager as you may be to get started, don't just leap out of bed and start

doing splits. Your muscles need to have some blood pumping through them, and be warm and at least somewhat supple to be stretched safely and effectively. Always warm up for a few minutes by running in place, jumping rope, or performing some light calisthenics before you start asking your muscles to lengthen.

2. No pain, period. It's tempting to try to speed your progress by stretching just a little bit further than is comfortably possible, but resist the urge to do so. Muscles are equipped with a safety mechanism called a stretch reflex. When you push a muscle too far, this sensor kicks in and the muscle responds with a reflexive contraction, shortening the muscle to protect it from overextending the joint. This is not the response you want when you're trying to lengthen tight muscles. Stretch only to the point where you feel gentle tension, then stop and hold the stretch. As you continue to stretch regularly, you'll be able to reach progressively farther and farther before you feel that tension. Becoming flexible means being able to stretch your muscles without pain.

3. Maybe before, definitely after. Most fitness professionals will tell you to stretch before and after any physical activity, which is great advice. But like most folks, you'll probably never do it. Stretching before exercise means taking 5 minutes to warm up, stopping and stretching, then resuming activity—something most people don't find practical. Plus, a recent study of more than 2,600 Army recruits found that, contrary to conventional wisdom, stretching before exercise didn't alter injury rate during activity. But stretching *after* exercising was still important to keep muscles performing at their optimal range of motion.

The take-home advice is to warm up at a light pace, gradually increasing your intensity and purposefully stretching out your movements to boost your circulation and get your muscles ready for activity. Exercise as normal. When you're done, cool down, then spend 5 to 10 minutes gently stretching the muscles you've just used before hitting the showers. It's a natural progression that'll leave you feeling great all over.

4. Slow and steady. Don't bounce while you stretch. This point has been repeated ad nauseum, yet some people are still locked into that "bobbing" and stretching mode. It's counterproductive and can cause injury. Keep your stretches slow and steady, holding each stretch 10 to 30 seconds.

5. Breathe. It sounds simple, but it's easy to forget. Breathe deeply during your stretches. If you find yourself holding your breath, you're pushing too hard.

6. Sneak it in. Ideally, you should stretch every day. If that's not realistic, at least stretch the muscles you use on the days you work them. You can make this a no-brainer by simply working your stretches into your routine. On weight-training days, for instance, stretch the muscles you're

working in between sets. So after a set of chest presses, stretch your pectorals; after squats, stretch your legs. It's a more efficient use of your time, and you'll lift better because your muscles are more limber.

Total-Body Flexibility

It's important to stretch the muscles you use most heavily. If you run, for example, you have to stretch your quadriceps, calves, and hamstrings. But it's also important to stretch the muscles you use less often. You may not use your chest muscles a great deal while you're sitting at your desk, but over time, that hunched-over position can leave them shortened if you don't make a conscious effort to stretch out. The fact that muscles and tendons naturally lose some of their flexibility as we age is all the more reason to do some full-body stretching 3 or 4 days a week.

Neck

four-direction neck stretch

Sit or stand with your back straight, your head in line with your spine, and your eyes facing forward. Let your arms hang naturally at your sides.

Slowly turn your head to the right as far as it will comfortably go (1). Hold the stretch there, then repeat on the left side (2). Return to the starting position. Slowly drop your head and tuck your chin into your chest until you feel a mild pull (3). Hold, then tilt your head upward until you are looking up about 45 degrees (4). (Do not rest the back of your head against your shoulders.) Hold, then return to the starting position.

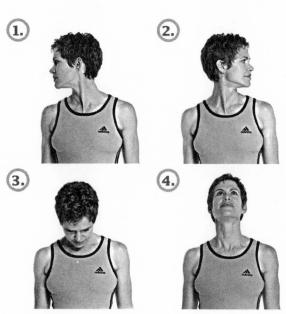

side-to-side stretch

Sit or stand with your back straight, your head in line with your spine, and your eyes facing forward. Let your arms hang naturally at your sides.

Slowly and gently allow your head to fall toward your right shoulder (1). Stop and hold when you feel a gentle stretch. Slowly bring your head back to the starting position, then do the stretch toward your left shoulder (2).

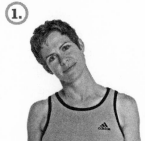
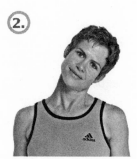

Shoulders

praise pose

Get down on your hands and knees, keeping your back flat, your neck straight, and your eyes facing toward the floor.

Slowly shift your weight backward so that your butt sits back on your heels and your arms straighten out in front of you. Try to keep your hands in their original position; do not allow them to shift back as you bend. You should feel a stretch in your arms, shoulders, and hips.

overhead reach

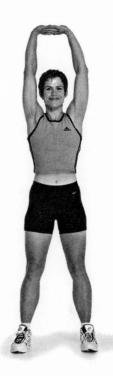

Stand with your feet hip- to shoulder-width apart, your head in line with your spine, your back straight, and your eyes facing forward.

Slowly and gently reach both arms directly over your head while keeping your eyes facing forward. Be careful not to arch your back. When your arms are directly overhead, lace your fingers together with your palms facing the ceiling. Hold, then return to the starting position.

Arms

back scratch stretch

Stand with your feet shoulder-width apart, your back straight, your head in line with your spine, and your eyes facing forward. Raise your left arm over your head, bend your elbow, and reach your hand down behind your head to the middle of your back. The fingers on your left hand should fall between your shoulder blades and your left elbow should point toward the ceiling.

Keeping your shoulders down, grasp your left elbow with your right hand and gently push the elbow down until you feel the stretch in the back of your arm. Hold, then return to the starting position and repeat with your right arm.

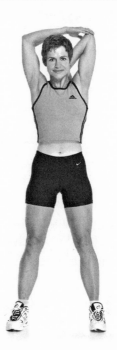

open arms

Stand with your feet shoulder-width apart and your knees slightly bent for support. Keep your back straight and your head up.

Slowly raise your arms up and out to the sides until they reach shoulder level. With your palms facing forward, gently pull your arms back behind you, keeping them just slightly below shoulder level. When you have pulled back as far as is comfortably possible, bend your wrists back until you feel a stretch in the fronts of your upper arms. Hold, then slowly return to the starting position.

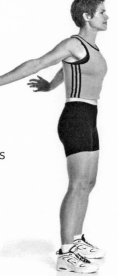

Chest

doorway pec stretch

Stand in a doorway with your feet shoulder-width apart. Lift your right arm and bend it at the elbow so that your upper arm is parallel to the floor and your fingers are pointed toward the ceiling. Press your hand and forearm against the doorway.

Slowly rotate your body toward the opposite shoulder, causing the arm against the doorway to be pulled back. You should feel the stretch across your chest and in your shoulder. Hold, then repeat with your left arm.

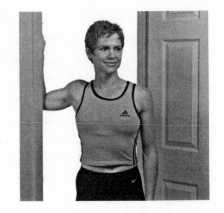

arms-back stretch

Stand with your feet shoulder-width apart and your knees slightly bent for support. Clasp your hands behind your back with your palms facing in toward your body.

Gently and slowly push your chest forward, keeping your back and abs stable as you stretch. Hold at the point where you feel your chest "open." Return to the starting position.

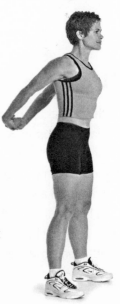

Upper Back

self-hug

Stand with your feet shoulder-width apart, your knees slightly bent for support, your head in line with your spine, and your eyes facing forward.

Wrap your arms around the front of your body as though you are giving yourself a hug. Grasp the backs of your shoulders with your hands. Keeping your torso steady, relax your upper back and shoulders and allow your head to hang forward as far as is comfortably possible. Hold, then slowly return to the starting position.

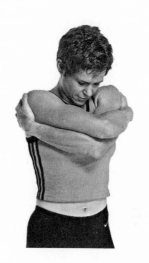

tabletop bend

Stand a few feet away from a sturdy table or countertop with your feet shoulder-width apart. Lean forward slightly and place both palms flat on the tabletop, positioned slightly wider than shoulder-width apart. Keep your knees soft.

Keeping your back straight and your shoulders down, bend forward at the waist until your arms and back are parallel to the floor. Push your head and chest gently toward the ground until you feel a stretch. Hold, then slowly return to the starting position.

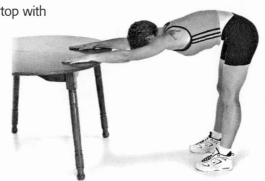

Lower Back

in-the-womb stretch

Lie flat on your back with your knees bent and your feet flat on the floor. (This is done most comfortably on a carpeted or well-padded surface.)

Keeping your head and shoulders on the floor, lift your legs and bend your knees up toward your chest. To increase the stretch, gently pull your knees farther toward your chest. Hold, then return to the starting position.

spine twist

Lie on your back with your arms extended out to the sides so that your body forms a T.

Keeping your shoulders flat on the floor, slowly bend your right knee up toward your chest and drop your bent leg across your body to the left. Turn your head to look down across your left arm. Hold, then return to the starting position. Repeat with your left leg.

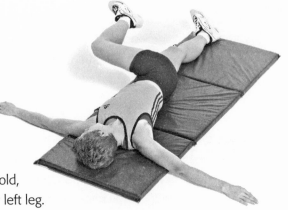

Hips

stair stretch

Stand facing away from a low chair or the bottom of a staircase. Carefully extend your right leg behind you, placing the top of your foot on the chair or on one of the lower stairs behind you. Place your hands on your hips, or hold on to a table or wall for support.

   Keeping your right foot securely in place, gently pull your right thigh forward so that you feel a mild pulling through your right hip and thigh. Hold, then return to the starting position. Repeat with your left leg.

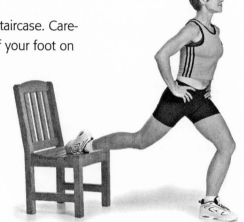

crossover leg pull

Lie on your back with your right leg bent at about a 90-degree angle and your right foot planted on the floor. Bend your left leg and cross your left ankle over your right knee.

   Clasp your hands behind your right knee and gently pull your right leg up toward you, keeping your left leg open and your left knee out to the side. Hold when you feel the stretch in your hip and inner thigh, then return to the starting position. Repeat with your left leg.

Abs and Obliques

cobra rising

Lie facedown with your hands on the floor directly under your shoulders.

Slowly and gently push into the floor with your hands and raise your upper body as far off the floor as you can by straightening your elbows and arching your back. Your hips should stay in contact with the floor. Your shoulders should be down in their natural position, and your chest should be out. Keep your eyes facing straight ahead. Hold, then lower yourself back to the starting position.

standing torso twist

Stand an arm's length away from a wall, facing it with your left side. Place your left hand on the wall.

Standing in place, reach your right arm across the front of your body, stretching your right hand toward the wall (it's okay if you can't touch it) until you feel the stretch in your torso. Hold, then return to the starting position. Turn around and repeat the stretch with your right arm.

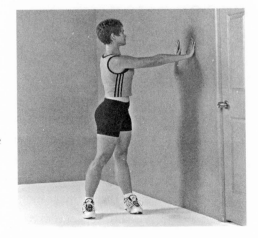

Quadriceps

stork stretch

Stand with your left hand resting on a chair or a table for support. Bend your right leg behind you and grasp the top of your right foot with your right hand, keeping your back straight and your eyes facing forward.

Slowly pull the heel of your foot toward your butt (not all the way up; that's a dangerous angle), stopping when you feel tension in your quadriceps. Be sure to keep your hips and knees aligned with one another. Do not lock the knee of your supporting leg. Hold, then return to the starting position. Repeat with your left leg.

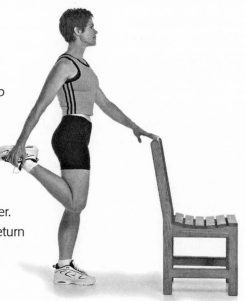

bench stretch

Lie on your back on a bench, an aerobic step, or the edge of a very firm, supportive bed with your right leg hanging off the edge.

Bring your left knee to your body and hold it with your left hand. Reach down and grasp your right ankle with your right hand, and slowly pull your right foot toward your butt until you feel the stretch in your quadriceps. Hold, then return to the starting position. Repeat the stretch with your left leg.

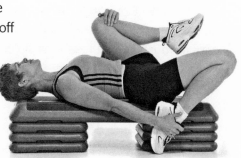

Hamstrings

leg extension and pull

Lie on the floor with your knees bent and your back flat. (This is done most comfortably on a carpeted or well-padded surface.)

Keeping both hips on the floor, slowly straighten your right knee and lift your right leg straight toward the ceiling with your foot flexed. Grasp your lower thigh and pull gently to increase the stretch. Hold, then return to the starting position. Repeat with your left leg.

To make this stretch more difficult, begin with both legs fully extended on the floor. Then bend your right knee up toward your chest, and slowly straighten it toward the ceiling.

sit and reach

Sit on the floor with your left leg extended straight out in front of you, your left foot flexed, and your right leg bent so that the sole of your right foot rests against your left inner thigh. Keep your back straight, your head in line with your spine, and your eyes facing forward.

Slowly and gently bend forward from the waist, running your hands down your leg toward your ankle and leaning over your left leg until you feel the stretch. Hold, then return to the starting position. Repeat with your right leg.

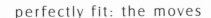

Groin

giant V

Lie flat on your back with your legs extended straight up above your hips and your feet flexed.

Slowly and gently allow your legs to open toward the floor. Place your hands on the inside of each knee and gently press until you feel slight tension in your inner thighs. Hold, then slowly return to the starting position.

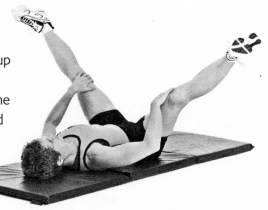

butterfly

Sit on the floor, bend your knees to bring the soles of your feet together, and drop your knees out to the sides. Keep your back straight, your head in line with your spine, and your eyes facing forward.

Place your hands around your ankles. Bend forward slightly, and using your forearms, gently press your knees toward the floor until you feel a stretch. Hold, then slowly return to the starting position.

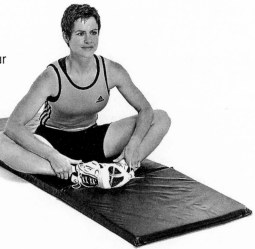

Calves

wall stretch

Stand an arm's length from a wall and place your palms flat against it.

   Extend your right leg 2 to 3 feet behind you and press your right heel to the floor. (Your left knee will bend naturally as you extend back.) Keep both heels flat against the floor. Hold, then return to the starting position. Repeat with your left leg.

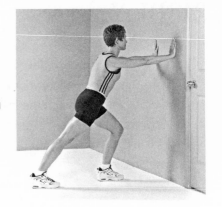

step stretch

Stand facing a step or a curb, with your legs hip-width apart and your back straight. Keeping your right foot flat on the ground, step forward with your left foot, resting the ball of your foot on the edge of the step and allowing your heel to lower to the ground. Slowly lean forward until you feel a stretch in your calf. Hold, then return to the starting position. Repeat with your right leg.

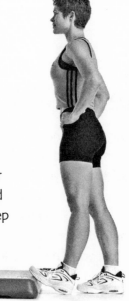

PERFECTLY FIT

the
system

choose the right program for you

How to make it happen

You have the gear. You've seen the exercises. Now you're ready for the programs. This is where you pull it all together and put your body through the paces. Waiting at the finish line are the ready-to-bare arms, butt, legs, abs, back, and chest you've been looking for. And you'll have the strength, coordination, and confidence to use them like never before.

The directions are very straightforward: Simply flip through and pick the program that best matches the fitness level you're at right now. If you're brand spanking new to the weight-lifting game, your best bet is to start out with chapter 21, aptly named Just Starting Out. This program will help you to build a base and tone your whole body.

If you're already active and have some strength-training experience under your belt, take a peek at chapter 22. It's specially designed to jump-start your muscles and make your weight-training work faster and better.

Have you been lifting for a while and are itching to put some serious buff on that tone? Then read chapter 23 for advanced exercise techniques.

And because women's glutes are often a problem area, the training program in chapter 24 has been specifically created to get your butt in swimsuit shape.

Fly, Baby, Fly

No matter at what level you start, there are programs to work and sculpt your body for practically the next year without ever repeating an exercise! Beginners will be able to climb their way up to the more advanced exercises, and seasoned lifters will find that with a little added weight, the beginner and intermediate programs are tough enough to make even their most well-formed muscles beg for mercy.

But don't stop there. You have more than 80 exercises at your fingertips, so why not create some of your own programs? Chapter 25 will show you how to string moves together to develop a killer program designed for your toning wants and fitness needs.

Finally, each program offers advice on the number of sets and reps for each exercise. These parameters will provide the best overall results for the majority of women. But ultimately, you're not limited to those parameters. You can always get clever and experiment with some of the set and rep combinations described in chapter 4, if only just for kicks. The variety will keep your muscles challenged and your mind having fun.

The number of programs you can develop and approaches you can take to your weight-lifting routine are endless. You've already taken the toughest steps by getting started. Now go on and enjoy your Perfectly Fit body for the rest of your life.

just starting out

16-week blastoff for beginners

Congratulations on your decision to get strong, fit, and toned. Even if you haven't done anything more strenuous than turning these pages, you've already done a lot more than most people do. You've gone from fantasizing about being fit to actually taking intelligent steps toward getting there.

If you've never strength trained before, I have some really good news for you. You're going to see results superfast. When women first start lifting, their muscle fibers have a lot of adapting to do, so they get firmer fast and tone up quickly. You'll feel stronger and notice some definition within 3 to 4 weeks. After 6 to 8 weeks, you'll start seeing clear improvements in your shoulders, arms, and lower body. And by the end of 16 weeks, entire muscle groups will be totally transformed.

Building a Better Body

Just because this is a beginner program, it is by no means an easy or wimpy routine. A seasoned strength trainer could still get a butt-kicking from it—she would just start out using more weight. The difference between this and the more advanced programs in this book is that this program includes more isolation exercises.

I'm a big fan of combination exercises that challenge your major, minor, supporting, and core muscles as well as balance and coordination all at once, but it would be plain stupid to start right out with those most challenging moves. New lifters usually have lots of muscle imbalances, as there are some muscles, like their

If I had just one tip to offer new lifters, it would be to focus. When you're going through a move, really concentrate on the muscles that are doing the work. Imagine them contracting to lift the weight and extending to lower it. Feel them getting stronger. Picture yourself lean, mean, and totally buff. When I first started lifting, I was considerably out of shape. I hated how blob-like I felt when I worked out, and I wasn't too crazy about the image staring back at me in the mirror. So instead of focusing on all the bad stuff, I focused on what I wanted to become. I loved feeling my muscles harden and watching previously flabby areas get firm. By concentrating on where I wanted to go, I got there faster and felt better about myself along the way.

as you push forward, pull back, and alternate your efforts between upper- and lower-body muscles. Notice how you are working through and strengthening each muscle group. You will feel stronger and more confident with every session.

Getting Started

Aim to do your strength-training routine 3 days a week. For the first few weeks, do one set of 10 to 12 repetitions for each exercise. Once you become comfortable, work up to two sets of 12 to 15 reps (you should be ready to progress to this next step by week 3 or 4). When you've completed the 16-week program, you have a choice. You can start at the beginning and repeat the sequence, using more weight this time. This will build a superstrong base. Or, if you're ready for a new challenge, you can move to the program in chapter 22, which is designed to challenge women with lifting experience.

legs, that they use all the time for everyday activity like walking; other muscles, like their triceps, get very little use. It's important to get all those muscles up to speed, using isolation exercises, before putting things together.

Because this is a progressive program, it builds your confidence as well as your muscles. You won't feel like you're getting thrown in the deep end before you know how to swim.

This 16-week workout is designed to get your muscles into the flow of strength training, starting with basic moves and working up to more complex Perfectly Fit–style exercises. Along the way, you should start feeling the rhythm of the workout

Quick Tips

✔ Warm up before you lift, and stretch when you are finished. This is the one step that even experienced lifters tend to blow off. The harder you work your body, the more important stretching is.

✔ Remember that something is *always* better than nothing. If you find yourself running short on time, do just one set of your exercises. You'll maintain your gains and won't fall out of your routine.

Weeks 1 through 4

The first 4 weeks of the program combine very simple combination exercises with basic isolation exercises. The goal is to develop a solid foundation of strength while smoothing out any muscular imbalances. You'll work your upper body first, leaving your legs fresh to support you during the moves. Then you'll hit the floor for lower-body work. You should feel more strong, stable, and balanced by the end of this block.

Wood chop
(p. 49)
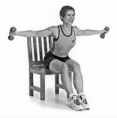

Dumbbell side swing
(p. 146)
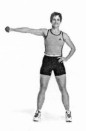

Dumbbell press
(p. 66)
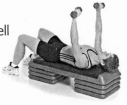

Seated back fly
(p. 68)
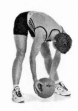

Lat pulldown
(p. 138)
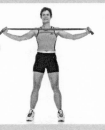

Simultaneous dumbbell curl
(p. 91)
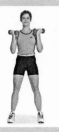

Behind-your-back arm raise
(p. 93)
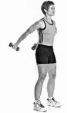

Seated straight-leg lift
(p. 114)
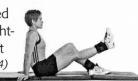

Lying leg curl
(p. 116)
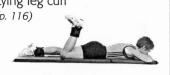

All-fours kickback
(p. 103)
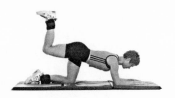

2-second floor crunch
(p. 126)
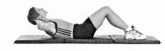

Weeks 5 through 8

Like weeks 1 through 4, the second block of this program combines basic combination exercises with isolation moves since you're still working on developing a solid strength and balance foundation. You'll be targeting the same muscles you worked during weeks 1 through 4 from different angles. This will help you challenge more muscle fibers and build muscle tissue (and consequently burn fat) more quickly. You should start seeing muscle definition and feeling significantly stronger by the end of this block.

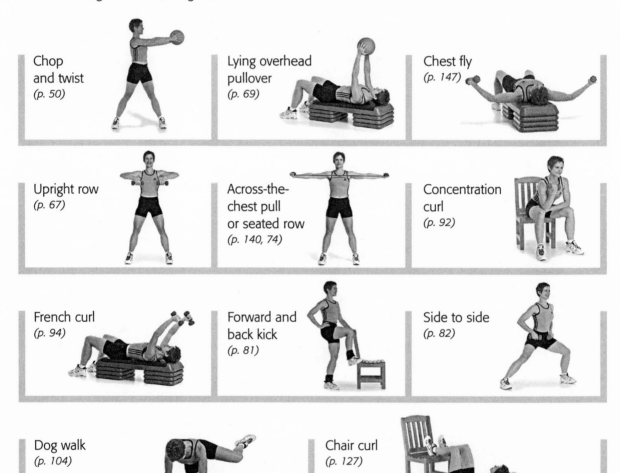

Chop and twist
(p. 50)

Lying overhead pullover
(p. 69)

Chest fly
(p. 147)

Upright row
(p. 67)

Across-the-chest pull or seated row
(p. 140, 74)

Concentration curl
(p. 92)

French curl
(p. 94)

Forward and back kick
(p. 81)

Side to side
(p. 82)

Dog walk
(p. 104)

Chair curl
(p. 127)

Weeks 9 through 12

After 2 months of solid strength training, your muscles are ready for some new challenges. This block still has you working your upper body first and your lower body last so that your big, strong muscles are fresh to support you. But a few slightly more advanced moves have been added to recruit any as-yet-unused muscle fibers and to further develop your core body strength. By the end of this block, once-strenuous tasks like carrying heavy bags of groceries should feel significantly easier, and you'll look better in your clothes to boot.

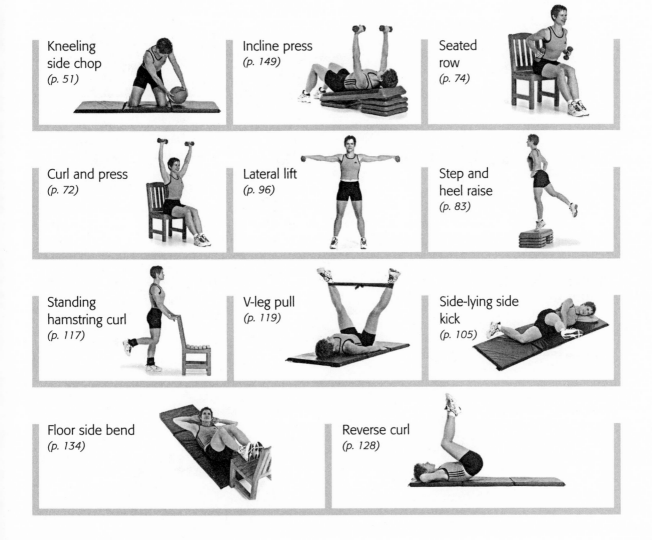

Kneeling side chop
(p. 51)

Incline press
(p. 149)

Seated row
(p. 74)

Curl and press
(p. 72)

Lateral lift
(p. 96)

Step and heel raise
(p. 83)

Standing hamstring curl
(p. 117)

V-leg pull
(p. 119)

Side-lying side kick
(p. 105)

Floor side bend
(p. 134)

Reverse curl
(p. 128)

Weeks 13 through 16

As you're no longer a true novice, your developing muscles are ready for some new challenges. During the final weeks of the program, you'll be adding a few combination moves that challenge your strength, coordination, and balance. They may feel a little tricky at first, but with your solid foundation, you'll master them in no time. By the end of this block, you'll be standing straighter and walking stronger, and you'll feel more confident and energetic.

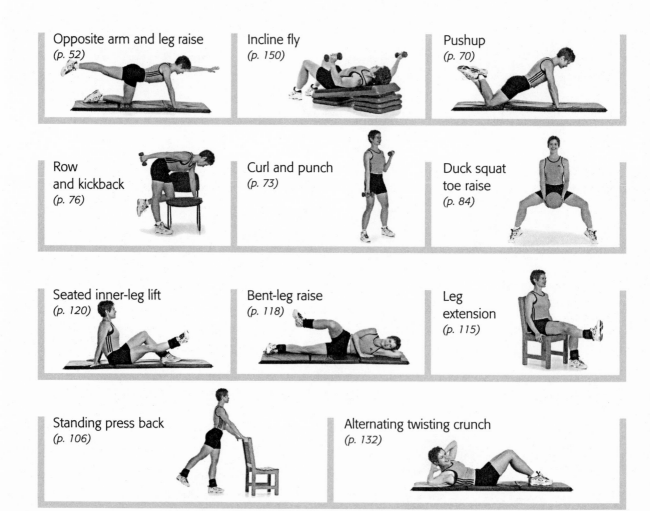

Opposite arm and leg raise
(p. 52)

Incline fly
(p. 150)

Pushup
(p. 70)

Row and kickback
(p. 76)

Curl and punch
(p. 73)

Duck squat toe raise
(p. 84)

Seated inner-leg lift
(p. 120)

Bent-leg raise
(p. 118)

Leg extension
(p. 115)

Standing press back
(p. 106)

Alternating twisting crunch
(p. 132)

off the plateau

8-week result revver for active women

There's nothing like the first several months of strength training. You're losing fat, gaining tone, and enjoying the payoff of sticking with your program as you zip your jeans and check out your reflection each morning. Then, when you're just about where you want to be . . . it all seems to stop working.

You're hoisting the same 10-pound dumbbells and pushing through the same routine, but while your body hasn't lost any tone, it hasn't gained any either. Or worse, some of that long-lost weight starts creeping back. What the *&^%???

That's what I thought when this happened to me a year or so after my introduction to strength training. Then I learned that the "*&^%" was more scientifically called the plateau. It's something we all hit at one time or another. It can sneak up on you a few months or even a few years after you start strength training—sometimes without your really noticing it. And if you don't find a way around it, you risk burning out and losing your hard-earned gains.

Past the Sticking Point

The science behind the plateau is actually pretty simple. What happens is that after a few weeks, your neuromuscular system steps up to the challenge of your routine. It can perform the work at hand without developing more mind-muscle connections or building more muscle fibers. At that point, you usually increase the weight you're lifting to give your muscles a fresh challenge. But this can only work for so long. At the point where you "max out" the amount you can lift, the plateau hits. And because you're not making any fresh muscle, you start burning fewer calories and seeing fewer results. To get off this plateau, you have to toss your body a curveball and challenge your muscles in some surprising new ways.

The best way to do that is with some total-body combination moves, which challenge your major, minor, core, and supporting muscles (as well as a few muscles you probably didn't know you have). And by all means, try this program even if you're feeling fit and not currently on a plateau. Expanding your repertoire is important to keep both your mind and your body challenged, to continue feeling jazzed about your workouts, and to continue developing muscle tone and definition. The following is an 8-week total-body blowout designed to open new neuromuscular connections, wake up bored muscles, and jump-start your muscle toning.

Getting Started

You should aim to do your strength-training routine 3 days a week. Because some of these exercises are a little more complex, it's a good idea to get the hang of the motion by trying them with a very light weight or no weight at all. When you have the movement down, add a little weight and give it a go. For the first few sessions, do just one set of 10 to 12 repetitions to give your muscles time to adapt to these new challenges. Once you

become comfortable (this shouldn't take more than a week or two), work up to two sets of 12 to 15 reps. When you've completed the 8-week program, you have a choice. You can start at the beginning and repeat the sequence, adding more weight to avoid the dreaded plateau. You can read chapter 23, which introduces some advanced toning techniques. Or, if you're feeling adventurous, you can go to chapter 25 and create your own routines.

Weeks 1 through 4

The first 4 weeks of this program include a wide array of combination moves to challenge your muscles, balance, and coordination. The goal is to hit your muscles from every possible angle in ways they haven't yet been worked before. By the end of this block, you should see improvement in your balance and total-body muscle tone.

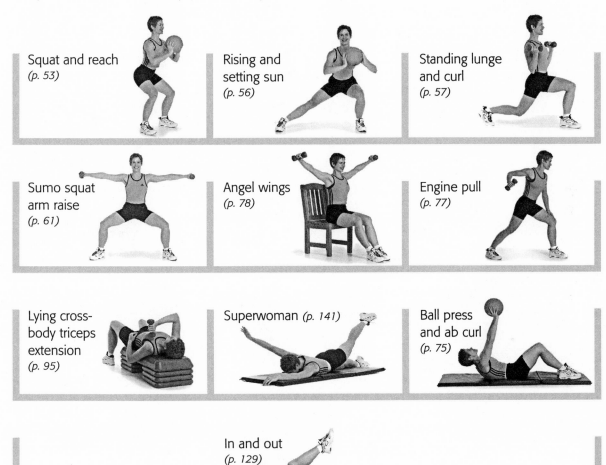

Squat and reach
(p. 53)

Rising and setting sun
(p. 56)

Standing lunge and curl
(p. 57)

Sumo squat arm raise
(p. 61)

Angel wings
(p. 78)

Engine pull
(p. 77)

Lying cross-body triceps extension
(p. 95)

Superwoman *(p. 141)*

Ball press and ab curl
(p. 75)

In and out
(p. 129)

Weeks 5 through 8

During the second block of this program, you take the same muscles that you worked in the first 4 weeks and put them through yet another routine chock-full of unique, challenging moves. Again, the idea is to work your body from every angle that you can. As a bonus, your core muscles (abs, back, hips) become finely strengthened and toned from supporting your body throughout these routines.

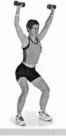

Dumbbell squat and upward press
(p. 54)

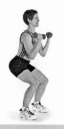

Curl and half-squat
(p. 59)

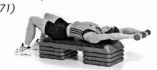

Synchronized kickback
(p. 62)

Rockette
(p. 85)

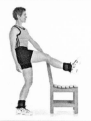

Rubber band sidestep
(p. 109)

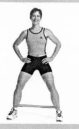

Arm raise pullover
(p. 71)

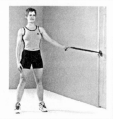

Single-arm crossover
(p. 148)

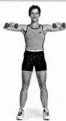

Water pitcher fly
(p. 98)

Sprinter start
(p. 60)

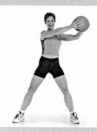

Ditch digger
(p. 58)

Hand-to-foot ball curl
(p. 130)

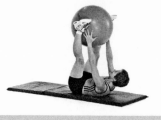

to the next level

Advanced toning techniques

Way to go, woman! Opening this chapter means you've been kicking butt and taking names long enough to feel strong, confident, and sexy. At this point, you've either successfully completed all of the exercises in the beginner or the intermediate chapter or you've spent some time following your own exercise routine. Either way, this is the perfect time to get up off those laurels you've been resting on and take your body to its outer limits.

This 8-week program is packed full of exercises that will challenge your balance and coordination as well as your major and minor muscle groups. Because many of these exercises involve using your upper- and lower-body muscles simultaneously, they also develop your core supporting muscles, which include your abs, obliques, and back. They also will finely chisel tough-to-tone areas like your obliques, outer glutes, and hips. But a tight butt and a serious six-pack aren't the end of the story (although I know some of you will argue otherwise). With a rock-steady core, you'll perform everything better. Your tennis serve will be faster, your karate-class high kicks will pack more power, and you'll swim, run, paddle, throw a Frisbee, and even walk swifter and stronger.

Getting Started

You should aim to do your strength-training routine 3 days a week. Because some of these exercises are a little more complex, it's a good idea to get the hang of the

between
YOU&ME

motion by trying them with a very light weight or no weight at all. When you have the movement down, add a little weight and give it a go. For the first few sessions, do just one set of 10 to 12 repetitions to give your muscles time to adapt to these new challenges. Once you become comfortable (this shouldn't take more than a week or two), work up to two sets of 12 to 15 reps for super body toning.

Note: A few exercises here—most notably the pullup, pushup, and chair dip—can be supertough, especially when you work up to doing the "full" version of these exercises. If you can't do 15 reps, do what you can, even if it's just 4 or 5. It will give you a goal to work toward, and you'll be stronger in the long run.

When you've completed the 8-week program, you have a choice. You can start at the beginning and repeat the sequence, adding more weight. You can also try some of the programs in the other chapters. Chapter 22 is filled with fun combination moves, and chapter 24 gives that lower body an extra boost. Or, you can go to chapter 25 and create your own routines.

Quick Tips

✔ Warm up before you lift, and stretch when you are finished. This is the one step that even experienced lifters tend to blow off. The harder you work your body, the more important stretching is.

✔ If you haven't worked with a medicine ball before, you may need an extra day of rest between workouts at first. Medicine balls challenge your muscles in a whole new way, and you'll probably be a little sore (in a good way) after the first few times you've used one.

✔ Remember that something is *always* better than nothing. If you find yourself running short on time, do just one set of your exercises. You'll maintain your gains and won't fall out of your routine.

✔ If you haven't already, take your strong, toned body outside and see what it can do. Go ride a bike. Shoot hoops. Or try your hand at a new sport. A sturdy, able (not to mention show-offable) body is your reward for hard work well done.

Weeks 1 through 4

The first block of this advanced program includes some challenging body-weight exercises such as the pullup. This is your chance to literally pull your own weight and to enjoy the tremendous body toning that these tough exercises provide.

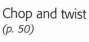

Chop and twist
(p. 50)

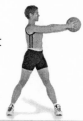

Ball swing knee kick
(p. 63)

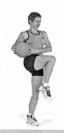

Lift, curl, and reach
(p. 65)

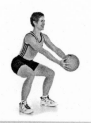

One-legged lunge
(p. 88)

Flamingo hip twist
(p. 110)

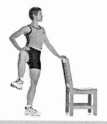

Pullup (modified or full)
(p. 79)

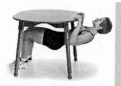

Reverse grip row
(p. 142)

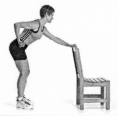

Pushup (full)
(p. 70)

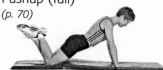

Lying cross-body triceps extension
(p. 95)

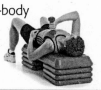

Concentration curl
(p. 92)

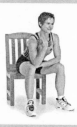

Circle crunch
(p. 135)

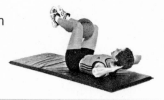

Weeks 5 through 8

Weeks 5 through 8 continue in the path of the first block, combining body-weight exercises with other challenging moves designed to fine-tune your balance, strength, and muscle tone. By the time you finish this block, you should feel like there is nothing you cannot do.

Kneeling side chop
(p. 51)

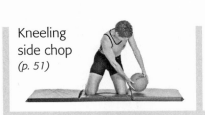

Squat and side lift
(p. 86)

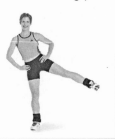

Lunge row
(p. 64)

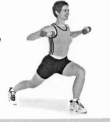

Side step and squat
(p. 87)

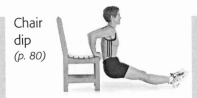

Step and extend
(p. 55)

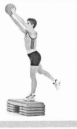

Alternating one-arm chest press
(p. 151)

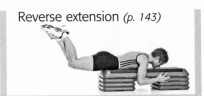

Chair dip
(p. 80)

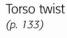

Arm raise pullover
(p. 71)

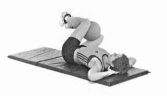

Reverse extension *(p. 143)*

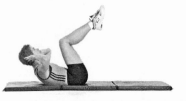

Torso twist
(p. 133)

In and out
(p. 129)

bikini-bottom jiggle blaster

8-week lower-body tone and go

Because we're women, our butts are the largest and potentially strongest of all of our muscles, giving us the power to get up and go as fast as our wandering feet will take us. They're also where we store excess fat to live off in times of famine. These days, however, we spend a lot more time sitting than striding. As a result, it's easy to end up with an ample bench cushion that is soft for sitting but isn't exactly an asset you want to show off at the beach.

So I've included a lower body–intensive program; even fit women sometimes need a little extra help back there. (I speak from experience . . . there's nothing like a three-way dressing room mirror to make you go, "Whoa!") If you have some extra "fuel" stored in your back cabinets, this program won't magically shed it. It will help, as you build muscle and burn more calories, but real fat burning is best done with consistent exercise and portion control.

If your muscle tone is mostly good but you just have some bikini-bottom jiggle, this glute-intensive workout will help firm and tone those muscles so that your cheeks stay a little steadier when you strut.

Many of the exercises in this program are borrowed from "dryland" routines that swimmers perform to put more power in their kick. (And they have some of the best butts in the business.) But to stay in line with the Perfectly Fit core-body

between
YOU&ME

toning philosophy, I've also included a few other exercises that will hit the upper body and the core muscles.

Even when you're concentrating on only one body region, you always want to maintain a balance of strength in all of your muscles. Besides, the more muscle fibers you build in both your upper and lower body, the better your metabolism will be at burning fat.

Getting Started

Aim to do your strength-training routine 3 days a week. Perform these routines as a circuit. That means you'll go through the whole routine once (one set of each exercise), then go through and do it again, with minimal rest (about 15 seconds) between the exercises. If you need to, you can rest for up to 2 minutes between the circuits. This will add an aerobic component to the routine and will help burn more calories and blast away more fat. Start with 10 to 12 reps of each exercise and work up to 12 to 15 reps. Start with one set and work up to three. I usually recommend only two sets of strength-training exercises, but running through this circuit three times will provide a longer cardio workout and optimum muscle toning.

Once you've completed the 8-week program, you have a choice. You can start at the beginning and repeat the sequence, adding more weight. Or you can go to chapter 25 and create your own routines, putting an emphasis on your lower body.

Quick Tips

✔ Warm up before you lift and stretch when you are finished. This is the one step that even experienced lifters tend to blow off. The harder you work your body, the more important stretching is.

✔ Remember that something is *always* better than nothing. If you find yourself running short on time, work through your circuit just once or twice. You'll maintain your gains and won't fall out of your routine.

Weeks 1 through 4

During this exercise block, you will combine lower-body squatting, extending, and lifting to challenge your glutes from every angle. By the end of the routine, your butt undoubtedly will burn, but it'll also feel firmer by the time you wrap up the fourth week.

Ditch digger
(p. 58)

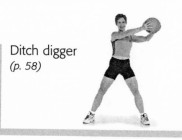

Squat and side lift
(p. 86)

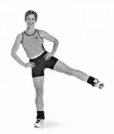

Bent-knee crossover
(p. 107)

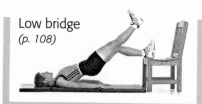

Low bridge
(p. 108)

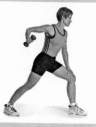

Rubber band sidestep
(p. 109)

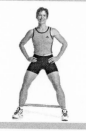

Side-lying side kick
(p. 105)

Leg extension
(p. 115)

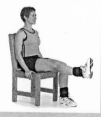

Single-arm crossover
(p. 148)

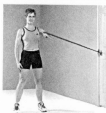

Curl and press
(p. 72)

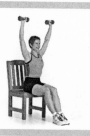

Engine pull
(p. 77)

Front arm raise
(p. 97)

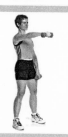

Floor side bend
(p. 134)

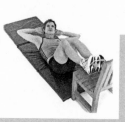

Weeks 5 through 8

The second half of this program introduces a new set of exercises to challenge your lower body in new ways so that you recruit different muscle fibers and boost your toning. By the end of this block, your butt and hips should feel higher and firmer, and they should appear more toned.

Rising and setting sun
(p. 56)
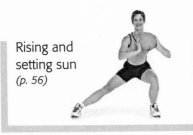

Step and heel raise
(p. 83)
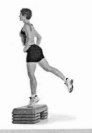

Standing press back
(p. 106)
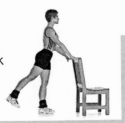

Lying inner-leg lift
(p. 121)
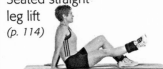

Monster walk
(p. 111)
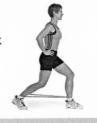

Dog walk
(p. 104)
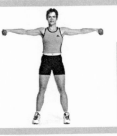

Seated straight-leg lift
(p. 114)
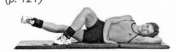

Pushup (modified or full) *(p. 70)*
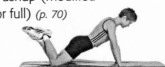

Lateral lift
(p. 96)
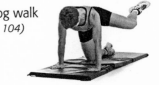

Seated row
(p. 74)
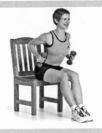

Partner ball toss (if you don't have a partner, do the alternating twisting crunch)
(p. 131, 132)
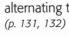
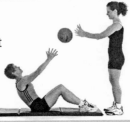

DIY programming

Try your hand at training

The programs in this book are 8 weeks long, except for Just Starting Out, which is 16 weeks long. That doesn't mean, however, that you can do those routines for just 2 months and then retire to the life of a buff-bodied diva. You have to keep it up. But you shouldn't just keep doing the same exercises over and over again. Your body and brain need regular change to maintain sharpness and tone.

The Right Mix

When you're ready to start creating your own programs, the trick is finding the right balance of exercises. Ideally, you want about 10 exercises that, when combined, will challenge all of your major muscle groups: back, chest, arms, legs, and abs. But you can also design programs that lean a little more heavily on the areas where you need the most toning. If your upper body tends to be weak, for example, you should concentrate more on arm, back, and chest exercises and a little less on the legs and butt. Generally, order your exercise routine so that you work the biggest muscles (like those in your legs) first, and the smallest muscles (like those in your shoulders) next. (Abs can go last.) Working through the programs in the book should give you a clearer sense of how exercises should be ordered. Your own program may eventually resemble the one shown on the sample journal page on page 191.

You also want to develop a routine that fits your fitness level. Each exercise in the book lists the muscles it works as well as an exercise rating that indicates

between
YOU&ME

Once you get the hang of it, designing your own programs is a total kick. Just one word to the wise: Always throw at least one exercise you don't like into the mix—because those are usually the ones that challenge you the most. When I first started lifting, I was following a coach's program that included these muscle-scorching "V-grip" pullups. I hated every moment of them. When I started designing my own programs, they were the first to go. Two years later, my back was noticeably weaker because I was blowing off exercises I didn't enjoy—like all the really tough back work. I've reluctantly started doing them again. I still hate them, but my back is toned and strong, and I don't get fatigued anymore from just sitting at my desk. The moral: Even if it sucks—especially if it sucks—do it. You'll be richly rewarded in the end.

whether it's a basic, intermediate, or advanced move. Remember that just because an exercise is rated as basic doesn't mean it can't give a killer workout to an experienced exerciser. Just use a little more weight to make it more challenging. Someone who is new to strength training would do best to start with basic to intermediate moves for the first few weeks, only because the more advanced exercises challenge your balancing and supporting muscles to a greater degree. These exercises are best done after you have built a foundation with the basics.

Finally, don't forget the Perfectly Fit philosophy. A strong core body means toned abs; a beautiful, straight back; great posture; and better performance in everything you do. Be sure to work in some total-body exercises from chapter 12. The following tips will help you get started.

Pick one of each. One of the easiest and most effective ways to build a program is to pick one exercise from each individual body-part chapter, such as arms in chapter 13, and one from each of the sections in chapter 12, Total-Body Toning. That way, you'll be sure to hit all of your major muscle groups, and you'll include a few upper- and lower-body combination moves to strengthen your core and stabilizing muscles.

Try a total-body blitz. Recreational athletes will benefit from performing a total-body blitz, especially during those months when they aren't working on their sport. To create a body-blitzing program, open up to chapter 12 and pick three moves from the total-body section, three from the upper-body moves, and three from the lower-body moves. Top it off with the ab exercise of your choice from chapter 16. You'll have a routine that puts your core and stabilizing muscles to the test while toning you up, burning fat, and improving your balance and coordination.

Have a ball or a bell or a band. The exercises in this book call for medicine balls, dumbbells, ankle weights, and exercise bands. Use these implements to get creative with your programming. Follow a routine of nothing but medicine ball exercises for 1 month. The next month do an exercise band program. The month after that, mix them all together. The only limit is truly your imagination.

JOURNAL PAGE

Exercise	Muscles worked	Sets	Reps	Weight (lb)
Rising and setting sun	Quads, glutes, deltoids, and triceps	1	10	5
Leg extension	Quads	1	12	3
Standing press back	Glutes	2	1	2
V-leg pull	Abductors	1	12	–
Dumbbell press	Pectorals, triceps, and deltoids	1	14	8
Incline press	Upper pectorals	2	12	6
Concentration curl	Biceps	1	15	6
Lying cross-body triceps extension	Triceps	1	12	5
Weighted shrug	Trapezius	2	10	5
Forearm extension	Forearm	1	10	3
Hand-to-foot ball curl	Rectus abdominis	2	10	–
Torso twist	Obliques	1	10	–

PART 4

PERFECTLY FIT

FIT

on the move

a body in motion

Burn fat, feel fabulous

When you want shapely muscles, strength training is second to none. But if you want to burn fat even faster while also revving your energy, busting your daily blahs, and lowering your risk of almost every chronic condition known to man, adding a few days of cardio activity into the mix is a must.

The basics of cardiovascular, or aerobic, exercise are simple. You use your body the way it was meant to be used—walking, running, jumping, and playing—and in return, your body looks and feels younger longer. Because cardio activities like swimming and cycling increase your endurance (meaning you can work and play longer without "bonking"), they're a perfect complement to resistance exercises, which make your muscles stronger. Taken together, strength training and aerobic exercise are the ultimate health and beauty tonic.

The Cardio Equation

Aerobic exercise is an activity that uses your major muscle groups and raises your heart rate for an extended time. It's called aerobic because your body needs more oxygen to fuel your efforts. But what few women understand is that it's the increased oxygen part that makes this activity so good for you.

You step out the door for a jog. As you pump your arms and legs, your brain sends a signal for you to breathe a little harder, which gets more oxygen into your system. As you inhale, the oxygen streams from your lungs into your bloodstream, where your heart can pump it to your working muscles. Your body then uses that oxygen to break down stored carbohydrates, fat, and protein into the energy that your muscles need to function. That fuel-making process burns calories—and fat.

If you keep your level of aerobic activity consistent, your metabolism will eventually change, too. Your body will be working, you'll burn more calories between workouts. Your heart and lungs will become more efficient at exchanging and carrying oxygen, so you'll be able to work out in the morning, work all day, and still have energy for a sexy night without feeling wiped out.

Give yourself 5 to 10 minutes to ease into activity and warm up and 5 to 10 minutes to cool down and stretch at the end, while allowing yourself a full 30 minutes of quality calorie-burning activity in between. If there are days when you can't block out 45 minutes, split the time and take a quick walk before and after work. Or if you can squeeze in just 20 minutes—do it. Something is *always* better than nothing.

It's probably easiest to do your aerobic workouts on alternating days with your strength-training workouts. If you do both workouts on the same day, do your strength training first so that your muscles are fresh. Then go and enjoy an easy-to-moderate cardiovascular workout. If you find that you need to do your aerobic exercise first, just use lighter weights for your strength-training routine.

The Calorie-Burning Cure-All

As if a revved-up metabolism weren't enough of a reward, research suggests that the more calories you burn through cardiovascular activity, the less likely you are to get cancer, heart disease, lung disease, stroke, depression, and diabetes. It may even fight the so-called fat gene. Here are just a few of the findings so far.

Get out of your genes. These days, scientists are as busy looking for a cure for obesity as they are for a cure for cancer. The funny thing is, they've probably already found it—in exercise. Remember all of the noise about the fat gene? It was a gene that manufactured a hormone called leptin, which is associated with obesity. Researchers hoped that if they could turn off this gene, they would have a miracle solution to obesity. Well, it turns out that regular exercise does the trick. Studies show that the equivalent of just 3 hours a week of jogging can drop leptin levels by 10 percent.

Lose the belly. Men naturally store their fat in their bellies. And as women reach their forties, they do, too. Blame it, along with those ice cream binges, on your hormones. But you can fix it (or prevent it) by changing your exercise habits. Research suggests that women who work out vigorously are less likely to gain fat around their middles than women who don't work out. Some researchers also believe that aerobic exercise specifically targets the layer of fat in the abdominal area. That's good news not only for your appearance but also for your health, since abdominal fat is associated with an increased risk for heart disease.

Get smarter, girl. It's no surprise that exercise is good for your brain, since it gives your gray

THE BIG CARDIO CALORIE BURN

Do you have weight to lose? Burn it off. Cardiovascular activity is best at burning calories, which lends a big helping hand to your weight-loss efforts. And if you're at the weight you like, it helps keep you there. Remember that 1 pound is equal to about 3,500 calories. Every few hundred calories you burn goes toward keeping unwanted weight off your waistline. Here's a snapshot of common cardiovascular exercises and how many calories the average 140-pound woman can burn during a 45-minute session.

Activity	Calories Burned
Bicycling (moderate)	382
Cardio kickboxing	334
Cross-country skiing	382
In-line skating (brisk pace)	334
Jogging	334
Rope jumping	477
Rowing machine	334
Snowshoeing	382
Stair-stepping machine	286
Stationary bicycling	334
Step aerobics	310
Swimming (freestyle)	382
Tennis (singles)	334
Trail walking	286
Walking (brisk)	310

matter a regular bath of freshly oxygenated blood, but the effects on your mental abilities are actually measurable. Researchers at the University of Illinois found that subjects who walked for about 45 minutes a day 3 days a week for 6 months scored 15 percent higher on tests that measured their ability to focus and perform multiple mental tasks than those who did a regular stretching program instead of working out.

Tone your heart. You've likely heard that regular exercise can lower your heart rate. But what does that really mean? Consider that in 60 seconds, a sedentary person's heart will beat 70 to 75 times—more than a beat per second. An active person's heart, on the other hand, is so strong that it can pump the same amount of blood in only 45 to 50 beats. That adds up to 36,000 fewer beats every day for fit women—13 *million* fewer at the end of just 1 year. Remember, your heart is the sole engine that powers your body. The easier it is for it to do its work, the longer it will keep on beating, and the healthier you'll feel.

Regular aerobic activity also lowers your blood pressure, cuts your bad cholesterol levels, and lowers your risk for stroke and heart disease. The results are measurable—and fast. When 12 overweight women started walking or stationary cycling for 1 hour each day, their blood pressures fell four points after just 1 week, according to researchers at the University of Pittsburgh in Pennsylvania.

Kick the blues. I can't count the number of times my mood was saved by a quick midafternoon run. It's amazing how the world can seem so dark and life so stressful at one moment, and so bright and airy just moments later as my first footfalls hit the pavement. Problems that once were overwhelming shrink down to a manageable size, and answers to previously complex dilemmas easily unfold. Even better, my mental outlook stays bright for the rest of the day. I'm not the only one who's experienced it, however. Studies have clearly shown that women who work out regularly are less likely to experience depression. And women who are mildly depressed almost always benefit when they start to work out.

Butt out. If I didn't exercise, I would smoke. I picked up the habit as a smart-enough-to-know-better high school girl. I was really sick of it by the time I graduated from college, but was hooked.

Cycling set me free. I loved riding with friends, but cigarette smoking kept me suffering behind them. Then I noticed that the more frequently I rode, the less I craved or enjoyed cigarettes. Eventually, I stopped smoking and started actually winning races. Do you need more proof? In a study of 280 women, researchers at Brown University found that women who quit smoking and started exercising were twice as likely to stay smoke-free and gained half as much weight as women who quit without exercising.

Close the fridge door. While it's common to feel a little hungrier once you start strength training, regular aerobic exercise helps tame your

THE PERFECTLY FIT RANGE

If you read enough about fitness, it won't be long before you come across recommendations for your "target heart range." This is the range, in the number of times your heart beats per minute, that fitness scientists say will yield the maximum fat-burning cardiovascular benefits while still being a sustainable effort.

To figure out your target heart range, you first determine your maximum heart rate by subtracting your age from 220. A 35-year-old woman, for example, would have a maximum heart rate of 185. Aim to work between 50 and 85 percent of that number. For the 35-year-old woman, that would be 93 to 157 beats per minute.

You can figure this out in one of two ways. You can invest in a heart rate monitor that will display your heart rate while exercising, or you can lightly lay your fingertips against your carotid artery and count the beats for 10 seconds and multiply your result by 6.

But I have a better idea. Instead of going to all that trouble, I recommend using a simple method known as your rate of perceived exertion (RPE). It's a math-free, expense-free way of knowing if you're working out hard enough. Studies have shown this method to be surprisingly accurate. Rate your efforts on a scale of 1 to 10, with 1 being chilling out on a chaise longue and 10 being running through a mud pit away from a fire. You want your workout to hover somewhere between 5 and 8. You should go hard enough so that you are breathing hard and exerting some effort, but not so hard that you're gasping for breath and praying for it to end.

As you get into better shape, you'll find that you'll be able to work out at a higher intensity (meaning you'll be moving more vigorously), yet still feel like you're in that 5 to 8 exertion range. That's how you know you're becoming fit.

appetite. It also helps to prevent you from eating out of boredom and frustration. When you become active, you start looking for physical activity, not food, to lift you out of a funk.

Outrun breast cancer. Breast cancer tops the list of almost every woman's most dreaded concerns. Population studies are finally revealing what scientists have suspected all along: Women who exercise regularly have a lower risk for the disease than their more sedentary counterparts. This is true even for women who started working out later in life, so it's never too late to get moving.

Your Perfect Cardio Fit

There must've been some magic in the running craze of the 1970s because even today, women have the notion that running is the only true aerobic exercise. Yes, running burns lots of calories per minute (about 9 per minute for a 140-pound woman). But if you haven't been jogging regularly, or you don't like running, every one of those minutes will feel like an eternity.

The real secret of a successful cardiovascular exercise plan is finding something you truly love to do. At the very least, you have to enjoy doing it. If it takes every speck of willpower just to get onto your stationary bike, you'll stop doing it within 6 months, and probably sooner. But if you actually look forward to your activity as a pleasant break in your day, you'll not only keep it up, but you'll also probably do more. Don't get me wrong; on some days it will still be tough to get moving. I love cycling, but when inertia has set in, it takes some internal nudging and nagging to get up and into my bike shorts. But I'm never sorry once I do.

between YOU&ME

It's great to find that one activity that really speaks to you, but don't limit yourself. When I first started cycling, I thought that was the only activity that counted. When I couldn't find time to ride, I'd be depressed. When I didn't feel like riding, I'd be depressed. Then it dawned on me that I needed to broaden my exercise repertoire. Now, if I don't feel like riding, I go for a run. It sounds simple, but I've seen lots of runners, swimmers, and kickboxing fanatics fall into the same trap. Keep your options open and be a well-rounded athlete. Both your body and your mind will thank you.

There is a fabulous array of exercise options available to women today—everything from African dance to sea kayaking. And of course, there's always walking, which is the most popular exercise among women. You'll find a wide selection of activities in this part, complete with instructions for getting started and tips on getting the most enjoyment and benefit from the activity.

If you're just starting out or getting started again after an extended layoff, have a little patience. No matter what activity you choose, the first few times out will probably be a little tough, especially if you've been very sedentary or are carrying extra weight. Don't give up. Do what you can, even if it's only 10 minutes. Your body adapts quickly, so it won't be more than a few weeks before you're feeling fitter.

the new fitness attitude

Goodbye stilted regimens, hello results

t happened again. A woman I know cornered me at a party. "I need help! I'm running 3 to 5 miles 4 days a week and lifting weights twice a week. And I'm not losing any weight!"

"How long have you been doing this routine?"

"Six months."

"And you've lost no weight?"

"Well, I did for a while. Then I hit a plateau."

"And you're still doing the exact same routine."

"Yes."

"That's the problem. Your body's bored. And you probably are, too."

It's a classic scenario. Women start a new routine and see quick, measurable results. But as their routine becomes *routine*, their bodies adapt, they push themselves a little less, and they stop seeing improvement. Before you know it, they grab a spoon and a pint and say, "To hell with it."

It's not their fault, really. The fitness industry is still young, and we made a few mistakes in our infancy—remember leg warmers and bouncing stretch routines? We also used to give people 10 strength-training exercises and told them to do 3 sets of 10 reps for eternity. If a woman worked out on a stair-stepping machine for 45 minutes 5 days a week, she was to be applauded, not questioned. We didn't appreciate the importance of variety, not only to prevent mental fatigue, but also to prevent muscle boredom.

We know better now. We know that while exercise consistency is important, infusing variety into our daily routines increases our strength and aerobic capacities faster than doing the exact same thing every day, with less likelihood of dropping out or injuring ourselves. It's also a whole lot more fun.

Muscle Mania

To understand the magic of cross-training, it helps to understand the metabolism of muscle building. When you challenge a muscle by bench-pressing a weight or pedaling a bicycle, it responds by first breaking down, then—with rest—building back up stronger and more solid. Those new and improved muscle fibers burn more calories and help you shed unwanted fat. As long as you keep riding farther or faster or lifting more weight, those muscles will continue to break down, build up, get stronger, and burn fat.

The problem is that you can ride only so far or bench-press so much weight. When you reach the point where you're going through the same motions at the same intensity, your muscles have adapted to the challenge. They stop getting stronger, and you burn fewer calories. How long it takes to reach this point depends on your current fitness level, but fitness scientists believe that

between YOU&ME

I discovered the real benefits of cross-training firsthand just a few years ago. After lifting weights and riding my bike day in and day out, I found that my fitness gains began to taper off and pounds started to creep on. Then I started triathlon training. As I swapped some of my time on the bike for long runs and morning swims, my body began to change. Twelve months later, I was 12 pounds leaner. Although I didn't work out more, I was lighter, stronger, and fitter at all of my sports than I had ever been at any one. Even if you love your exercise routine, your body will love it even more if you take a break from it.

muscles begin to adapt to repetitive movements in just 2 to 4 weeks.

That doesn't mean you have to start from scratch, dumping exercises and activities you really love every 4 weeks just to keep trim and toned. But tweaking your routine with intervals, cross-training, and new sets and reps will keep the results coming.

Daily Variety

One of the biggest reasons women fall into a routine and never come out is because that routine is easy. You know how, when, and where you run your 3.5 miles, so it's a no-brainer. Here are some equally easy ways to exercise your options.

Listen to Mr. La Lanne. I once interviewed Jack La Lanne, and the one tidbit I took away was, "When you don't have to think about what you're doing, it's time to do something else." He recommends changing your weight-training routine every 3–4 weeks, even just slightly, like doing arm curls with a barbell instead of dumbbells.

Aim for balance. When adding new activities to your cardio routine, aim for a balanced body. If you're Spinning on Mondays, try in-line skating on Wednesdays to challenge your leg muscles in a different way. Mix high-intensity activities like kickboxing with low-intensity exercise like yoga. The more muscles you can work from different angles in different ways, the more effective your exercise routine will be.

Include some mini-bouts. Don't forget that everyday activities count. Window washing, dog walking, taking the stairs, and daily stretch breaks breathe life into a stale routine, and even these small activities boost your calorie burn.

Try 'em all. Try one new activity a month. Or include a sample of activities every week. A killer cross-training week might look like this.

Monday: Total-body strength-training routine and an easy trek through the neighborhood

Tuesday: Spinning or outdoor cycling at high intensity for 45 to 60 minutes

Wednesday: Total-body strength-training routine and hatha yoga session for stress relief and stretching

Thursday: Thirty minutes of running, either outdoors or on a treadmill, adding hills or sprints for more intensity

Friday: Total-body strength-training routine and in-line skating at moderate intensity for 30 to 45 minutes

Saturday: Something fun and active for an hour or so

Sunday: Walk to ice cream shop for a sweet reward

kick-butt aerobics

More fun, more power, better body

Finally, someone has tapped into the power women have been channeling ever since Rosie the Riveter told them, "We can do it!" They tossed aside the tired conventional wisdom that girls just wanna dance and started offering up some serious kick-butt workout classes inspired by nothing less butt-kicking than the martial arts themselves.

You know the classes I'm talking about—Tae-Bo, cardio kickboxing, Aeroboxing, and Karate Integrated (KI) Aerobics, just to name a few. They've inspired droves of women, many of whom would never take a typical aerobic dance class, to punch, kick, shout, and let it all out—even if it's just in front of their TVs.

These classes are so popular, in fact, that women now make up the majority (56.5 percent) of participants in the once male-dominated discipline of kickboxing. If you haven't tried one of these powerhouse workouts yet, they're definitely worth a shot. They're one of the few aerobic activities that engage your mind, your body, and your spirit all at the same time.

Getting Started

All you need to get started is a supportive pair of shoes (any aerobics or cross-training shoe will do). For the more social at heart, I recommend calling around for

between YOU&ME

I usually tell women to leave their work troubles and relationship woes behind when they step out to exercise, but not with these ass-kicking cardio classes. Bring your anger with you and use it as fuel for those punches, jabs, and kicks. By the end of the class, you'll feel emotionally cleansed. And it beats ranting and raving at your boss.

classes at your local workout facilities. Some martial-arts studios offer these fitness classes in the evening, so you don't have to pay a gym fee to take them. If the workout-class scene isn't your bag, however, there are dozens of martial arts—inspired workout videos on the market.

Your biggest concern when choosing a class, whether live or a VHS version, is finding one that matches your fitness level. Martial-arts aerobics classes can be pretty high in intensity. So if you dive right into an experienced class, you run the risk of feeling frustrated and unfit before you throw your first jab-punch combination. Shop around for an entry-level class or videotape. And if you take a live class, let the instructor know that this is your first class so she can give you some pointers.

A typical class lasts about 50 minutes and follows a sequence of a gradual warmup, a jamming aerobic workout filled with butt-blasting kick-and-punch sequences, and a cooldown that includes some stretching and floor work. Aim to work out on 3 nonconsecutive days a week.

Tips and Techniques

Martial arts cardio workouts are centered on technique. Once you have the moves down, the rest is nothing but a heart-pumping groove. The following tips will help you to get started on the right foot.

Go easy on your joints. Some instructors will offer hand weights or dumbbells for you to use during the class. But don't use them; throwing punches with weights puts your joints at risk and is overly fatiguing, so it's easy for your form to fall apart. Keeping your punches and kicks in control will also protect your joints. Don't kick higher than is comfortable. And always keep your knees and elbows slightly soft when throwing kicks or punches.

kick-butt aerobics stats

Here's what you get from **50 minutes** of punching and kicking.

Calories burned
371 (based on a 140-pound woman)

Muscles worked
Pectorals, triceps, obliques, deltoids, and total lower body

Psychological benefits
You feel strong and confident while pummeling away daily stress. It's a kick to learn new skills.

BRUSHING UP ON THE BASICS

At first glance, all those kicks and punches can look pretty complicated. But if you pay close attention, you'll see that they're nothing more than a few basic moves put together in different combinations. Here are a few of the most common kicks and punches you'll be using.

❏ **The jab.** Stand with your left foot about a stride-length in front of your body and angle your body so that your left hip is turned slightly to the right and your body is at a diagonal angle. Come up on the ball of your right foot. Bend your elbows and hold your hands parallel to each other, fists in front of your face. To jab, push off your right foot, lean forward slightly, and extend your left arm straight from your body, turning your fist head-on as you do. Recoil by reversing the motion back to the starting position.

❏ **The punch.** The punch most often follows a jab or two. After you recoil from a jab, immediately push off your back foot, rotate your hips to the left, and extend your right arm, turning your fist head-on as you do. Recoil.

❏ **The uppercut.** Stand facing forward with your legs slightly wider than shoulder-width apart, your toes forward, and your knees slightly bent. Keep your fists up by your face. All in one motion, push off your right foot, rotate your right hip inward, and sweep your right arm down and up, bringing your fist up as though you are aiming for an opponent's chin. Recoil.

❏ **The hook.** Stand facing forward with your legs slightly wider than shoulder-width apart, your toes forward, and your knees slightly bent. Keep your fists up by your face. Push off your left foot, rotating your left hip inward, and bring your elbow up and out, sweeping your fist in a horizontal hook, as though aiming for an opponent's cheekbone. Recoil.

❏ **Knee kick.** Stand facing forward with your legs slightly wider than shoulder-width apart, your toes forward, and your knees slightly bent. Lift your right knee up to hip height, with your toes pointed down. Keeping your abs tight, extend your leg out in front of you and lean back slightly for balance. Recoil.

❏ **Side kick.** Stand facing forward with your legs slightly wider than shoulder-width apart, your toes forward, and your knees slightly bent. Lift your right knee up to hip height, with your toes pointed down. Pivot on your left foot as you lift your bent leg out to the side and extend it as though kicking your heel at an opponent's torso. Recoil.

Loosen up. Take a fashion tip from real martial artists and wear clothes that you can move in. Clothes that are cool and made of moisture-wicking fabrics are also a good idea since you'll heat up fast.

Drink up. Some instructors offer drink breaks before you hit the ground for floor work. If you don't want to run to the fountain or the refrigerator, just keep a water bottle handy for a quick sip when you need it.

bicycling

A bicycle built for you

Back in the old days, riding a "girl's bike" meant tooling around on a pretty painted bike that had a sloping top tube (just in case you wanted to ride in a long skirt) and a basket with a big plastic daisy on the front. Baby, have we come a long way.

Today, "girls" are tearing it up on a whole new breed of women-specific bikes that are built to suit their needs. Women's bikes have smaller frames to match our smaller statures, shorter brake levers for our smaller hands, flared saddles to accommodate our hips, and proportions designed to fit our torsos, arms, and legs so that we can ride faster, longer, and in comfort. Women can choose from road bikes, mountain bikes, touring bikes, or hybrids of different styles. And they still come in pretty colors. So if you haven't been on a two-wheeler since Santa brought you one for Christmas, now is definitely the time to take one out for a spin.

Yes, I'm biased. I race bikes and I love them. But there are reasons for that; I've seen more women of all ages (including yours truly) empowered by cycling than by almost any other sport. Pedaling down a rural road or through a city park rouses your spirit and awakens your senses. And it's hard to hate your thighs as you gleefully pull into the driveway after conquering a challenging ride.

Cycling is also a community sport, so you'll make new friends as you get into the best shape of your life. People who ride love to share their favorite routes with others and regularly plan outings to cool new places to ride. And single ladies, there are roughly a billion unattached bike-riding men looking for mates.

As if that weren't enough, cycling is as gentle on your body as a sport can be. There's a saying in sports medicine circles: Even if you can't run, walk, or hobble, you can ride a bike. Because cycling isn't a weight-bearing exercise, it's supereasy on your joints—even the achy ones. So it can be a wonderful, pain-free way to get exercise and lose weight.

If you're not sure you're ready to take the cycling plunge, try a Spinning class at your local Y or health club. This indoor-cycling workout is made to mimic outdoor riding. You'll burn about 500 calories during a 50-minute session. And it can get you in shape and juiced up to go out and try the real thing.

Getting Started

If you want to start riding, you need a bike. Like many women, you probably have one stashed away in the garage. Dust it off and look it over. Unless it's a pile of rust, it's probably ridable. Take it to a bike shop and have the parts replaced that wear out with disuse, like tires, inner tubes, cables, and the chain. For about $50, the in-house mechanic can lube it up and give it a little tender loving care, and you'll be ready to ride.

If you don't have a bike, don't worry. For a couple hundred bucks, you can be sitting pretty on a quality bike with sturdy parts and components. Even though you can buy a bike from just about any discount department store, I strongly recommend going to a bike shop instead. The folks

bicycling stats

Here's what you get from **60 minutes** of pedal power.

Calories burned
509 (moderate effort, based on a 140-pound woman)
Muscles worked
Glutes, quadriceps, hamstrings, gastrocnemius
Psychological benefits
It's a kick to get on your bike and go somewhere. Riding just makes you feel like going, "Whe-e-e-e-e!"

there know and love bikes. They'll measure you so that the bike you buy is sure to fit comfortably. They'll provide you with a warranty, and will often fix minor problems for free if you bought the bike there. So you're not overwhelmed by the selection when you walk in the door, here are the basic bikes you have to choose from.

Road bike. Characterized by skinny tires and a drop handlebar (it curves under), road bikes look a lot like the old 10-speeds you may remember, but these bikes have more gears and less weight, and are built for speed. If you aspire to long rides across the countryside and want to ride to your fullest potential, this type of bike is for you. The downside is that they're not designed to be cushy. Spending long rides bent over an aerodynamic handlebar takes some getting used to.

Mountain bike. The fat-tired cousins of the road bike, mountain bikes have a flat handlebar and beefier bodies. They're designed to cruise over roots and rocks on mountain trails, but they're also fun to ride on smooth dirt roads or in paved parks. Because they're so stable, they're easier to balance on than road bikes. If you plan on riding on dirt or through parks, a mountain bike is a good choice. The downside is that they're not as fast as road bikes either up- or downhill.

Cruiser or hybrid. Whether you call them cruisers, hybrids, or comfort bikes, these steeds all have one thing in common—they're practical. These are touring-around-town, beach-and-board-walk-loving bikes that emphasize comfort over speed. If you want a bike to trek to the store and to take with you for tooling around on vacations, cruisers are for you. The downside is that they're not well-suited for either serious road or off-road riding.

Once you have your bike, there are just a few accessories you'll want for your rides. Here's what to toss in your shopping cart.

Helmet. About 85 percent of head injuries can be eliminated by strapping on a helmet, which makes this accessory a must-have. A quality lid can cost as little as $30 and you can even buy one with a built-in ponytail holder.

Shorts. Bike shops can sell you padded Lycra shorts designed to keep your butt and other sensitive areas comfortable while spending long afternoons on a bike saddle. A good pair doesn't have to be expensive—about $35 or so—and they'll enhance your enjoyment of the ride. You can also buy padded brief underwear for about $20 at a bike shop. I like these because you can slip them on under any of your favorite shorts.

Gloves. While cycling gloves are not an outright necessity, they are a definite nicety, especially

if you plan to ride for more than an hour. They're padded to make a nice buffer for your hands when you're on bumpy roads, and are available for about $15.

Repair kit. A minipump, some extra tire tubes, and a patch kit are a wise woman's accessories. Chances are you won't need them very often, but you'll be glad you have them if you do need them. Ask the folks at the bike shop how to use them if you're unsure.

Bottle and bag. You'll want a water bottle to keep yourself hydrated and a little saddle bag (a bag that attaches to the back of your seat) to stash snacks, your repair kit, and emergency money for long rides.

If cycling becomes your sport, aim to ride about 4 days a week. Beginners should start out with 30-minute jaunts on flat terrain for the first 3 to 4 weeks. More experienced riders can add hills to their rides and can also include some long rides on the weekends. Make everyday rides more spirited by racing to street signs. Keep it fun.

Tips and Techniques

There's a saying that once you learn, you never forget how to ride a bike, and that's true. The motion and balance come back to you in a snap. But why stop there? Here are a few pointers that will make you stronger and more sure in the saddle.

Get in gear. Gears are wonderful inventions. They allow you to ride up hills without getting off and pushing, and to pedal fast on flat terrain. But learning proper shifting takes practice. A good rule of thumb is to be in a gear that allows you to pedal fairly quickly and easily so that your leg muscles don't wear out too soon. When you're riding on flat terrain, use the higher (larger) gears. As the terrain inclines, shift into lower (smaller) gears so you can keep pedaling at a steady cadence.

Practice pedaling. Many new bikes come with toe straps that hold your foot to the pedal. Some women are leery of being strapped to their bikes, but you'll love how easy the straps make pedaling once you get used to them. With them, you can produce pedaling power on the downstroke, when you push on the pedal, as well as on the upstroke, when your foot is circling back around. Good pedaling is an art among cyclists. Ultimately, you want to push and pull equally with both feet so that the pedals keep rotating in smooth, efficient circles.

Recruit new muscles. Long rides, especially hilly ones, can be fatiguing. One way to make them less so is to shift your weight on your bike to use "fresh" muscles when you need them. On little hills, shift your weight back to use your butt muscles. Shift forward slightly on the flats to maximize the use of your quads. Stand on steep hills to stretch out your legs and use your quads, hamstrings, and glutes at a different angle.

Go out with a group. When I first started riding, I was terribly intimidated about riding with other people. Now, I wouldn't have it any other way. Most bike shops organize rides or have information about organized rides, which are often to coffee shops on weekend mornings. No matter what your ability, you'll meet other riders just like you. When you ride and chat with others, the miles whoosh by faster, and you ultimately motivate each other to become fitter, faster riders.

running

The all-around sport

Maybe it's the simplicity. Maybe it's the camaraderie. Maybe it's the fact that almost no other sport gives you more overall body toning and calorie burning per minute. Whatever the reason, the sport of recreational running is attracting more women every year. In fact, women are far and away the fastest growing segment of new runners. As a result, there have never been more women-specific running events, running books, magazines, and Web sites as well as choices in running attire. If you used to run, like to run, or think you'd like to run, there's never been a better time to get going.

Probably the biggest advantage to taking up running is that it can be done practically anywhere, which is a huge draw for busy women. If you have a half-hour free from work and kids, lace up your shoes, head out the door, and you can get in all the exercise you need for the day. Running is also meditative, so it gives you a rare opportunity to collect your thoughts. And few forms of exercise tone your body as well. Even slow running uses more than 500 calories an hour, so you burn up those fat stores in a big way.

You keep burning those stores even when you're not running. Research shows that older women runners didn't have the same age-related slowdown in metabolism as their sedentary counterparts. Instead, the women who ran burned about 600 calories a week (almost 10 pounds a year) more, while the women who stayed sedentary gained weight. And it's never too late to take up this sport. Plenty of women start running in their forties and fifties; I know some women who didn't run their first marathons until they were 55 years old.

Getting Started

One of the great things about running is that you don't need much in the way of equipment. The two most important items are good running shoes and a bra that will keep your breasts from bouncing while you run.

Shoes. Because your feet are absorbing your body weight and propelling you off the ground, you *don't* want to skimp on your shoes. Fortunately, the technology has improved by leaps and bounds, and you can get a quality pair of shoes to fit your specific running needs for $50 to $100. Here's what to look for.

❒ **Fit.** I was 30 years old before I discovered that running shoes could actually be comfortable. I have flat, frog-flipper feet that always felt squished by the running shoes I bought at the mall stores. I thought it was normal to be in pain by the end of a long run. Wrong! Go to a running-specific store, have the salesperson measure your feet, and try different brands until you find a pair that fits perfectly out of the box. They should be wide enough to fit comfortably across your foot, and you should be able to wiggle your toes freely. They should be long enough so there's a thumb's-width distance between your longest toe and the end of the shoe.

running stats

Here's what you get from **30 minutes** of running.

Calories burned
318 (At a 10-minute mile pace, based on a 140-pound woman)

Muscles worked
Hip flexors, quadriceps, hamstrings, glutes, gastrocnemius, and to some degree, abdominals

Psychological benefits
Runner's high is real. Big troubles seem smaller; bad days become good days. And you have a sense of doing something perfectly healthy and natural for your body.

❒ **Terrain-specific.** If you plan to stick to the sidewalks around your neighborhood, look for running shoes with a thick, shock-absorbing sole. If you want to run on hiking trails, choose an all-terrain trail-running shoe that will offer more heel and ankle support. A knowledgeable salesperson can steer you toward the right makes and models.

Socks. Smart runners wear the socks they plan to run in when they shop for running shoes. An even better idea is to pick up some new running socks while you're shopping for your shoes. Most of us grew up running in white cotton gym socks; those things are a blister's best friend. Today, you can buy comfy acrylic or polyester running socks that stay drier than cotton and don't bunch up in your shoes. Happy feet make for happy runners.

Bra. If you're anything larger than an A cup, your breasts will bounce when you run. Small- to medium-breasted women can get by with a compression bra, which presses the breasts against the chest. But larger-breasted women find that a compression bra doesn't offer enough support. For C cups and beyond, the bra to try is the Champion Action Shape Bra, which won accolades in an American Council on Exercise review. This two-layer bra has an inner encapsulation layer to hold each breast firmly in place and an outer compression layer to provide backup bounce protection and give it a hip, casual look that can be worn without a shirt.

Your goal is to run 3 to 5 days a week. Beginners should start slowly, running only for as long as is comfortable, aiming for about 20 minutes. After a few months, you can work up to running 45 minutes at a stretch, but you should give your body a full rest 2 days a week.

Tips and Techniques

In some ways, running is the most natural activity in the world. As soon as we could walk, most of us took off as fast as our little feet would carry us. But in other ways, running is a little unnatural. Even as kids, most of us didn't keep chugging along for miles at a time. It takes a little practice and patience to condition your body for fitness running, but it's well worth the effort. The following tips can help.

Walk before you run. If you're brand new to running or just coming back after a long layoff, it will take a few weeks for you to work up to steady running. There's no shame in that. The trick is to not get discouraged when you have to stop running and catch your breath. Simply make it part of your training. The first few times out, wear a sports watch, and alternate between walking and running. Start out walking for 30 seconds to 3 minutes, then run for 30 seconds to 3 minutes. Repeat for about 30 minutes. You'll gradually stretch the amount of time you can spend running until you find you don't need to walk anymore.

Run tall. There is no "proper" running form, but there is good running form. Stand tall when you run, focusing your eyes about 25 feet in front of you. Hold your hands in loose fists and let your arms swing naturally at waist to chest level. Your stride should feel comfortable, not too short or too stretched out.

Take your time. It's natural to want to know how far you've run. But for fitness purposes, the distance isn't really as important as the time you spend running. Focusing on time also makes your workouts easier. Instead of worrying about mapping out a route of so many miles, just head out your door and run in one direction for 15 minutes (more or less, depending on your fitness level), then turn around and head home. It's that easy.

Go past the pavement. Running on nature and hiking trails is easier on your joints and tendons, and you can enjoy the scenery. If there are no nearby trails, check out your community parks and college campuses. They often have soft, cindered paths that are a joy for your joints and your eyes.

Avoid injuries. You can get too much of a good thing. High-mileage women runners are susceptible to knee, hip, and tendon problems. Avoid injury by taking rest days each week and mixing

between
YOU&ME

Running has helped me and many of my friends through the toughest periods of our lives. Whether it's getting fired or being dumped, it seems that there are no demons you can't outrun. It's cheaper than therapy, and it makes you feel better about your body, too.

your running with other activities like bicycling, swimming, and of course, strength training.

It's also *essential* to stretch after you run. Because of the impact and intensity, running can tighten those leg muscles more than any other kind of exercise. Always take 5 to 10 minutes to stretch your legs and your back after you've finished running.

Ease up. You'll build a better fitness base and be less likely to get sidelined by burnout or injury if you progress gradually. As a rule, you shouldn't increase your time or distance by more than 10 percent a week. So if you're currently running 30 minutes a day, 4 days a week, then you should add only 12 minutes to your total weekly running time the first week you increase.

Go for the T-shirt. Once you can run for 30 minutes without stopping, you should sign up for a 5-K (3.1-mile run). Don't worry; most runners at these "races" aren't competitive. They're there for the free T-shirt and to have some fun, just like you. These events help keep you motivated to run, and they leave you with a great sense of accomplishment when you cross the finish line.

cardioresistance training

Two workouts wrapped up in one

f you're the kind of woman who lines her lips and brushes her brows in the rearview mirror en route to work so as not to waste a precious second, this is the workout for you. Cardioresistance (CR) training—so named because it combines cardiovascular exercise with strength training—keeps your heart rate where it would be during an aerobic workout while you're doing your strength training. That means you get the cardiovascular fitness of a traditional aerobic workout and the lean muscle of a traditional weight-training workout in half the time it would take you to do both.

Developed and tested by fitness scientists at Ithaca College in New York, this technique is as effective, and in some cases more effective, for weight loss than traditional separate strength-training and aerobic exercise plans—most likely because it is less time consuming, so women stick with it.

Because CR training is a little intense, it might not be something you feel like doing every day. But if you're pressed for time, it's a great way to squeeze all of your exercise for the day into one jam-packed 45-minute session. And it can be a fresh change from your regular routine.

Getting Started

The technique is simple. You start with the list of strength-training exercises that you typically perform. But instead of resting between sets as you normally would, you get up and do an aerobic activity of your choice, such as jumping rope or riding a stationary bike. That way, when you've completed all the exercises, you're done with both your aerobics and your strength training for the day.

For example: Say the first two exercises on your routine are the Sumo Squat Arm Raise (page 61) and the Synchronized Kickback (page 62). You would perform your squats for 10 to 15 reps, then immediately begin an aerobic activity of your choice and perform that for 2½ minutes. When that time's up, you would move on to your set of kickbacks, followed by another 2½ minutes of aerobics. Continue like that until you have completed all your strength-training exercises. The whole routine takes 40 to 45 minutes (20+ minutes of cardio and 20+ minutes of strength training) to finish.

Tips and Techniques

CR training may feel awkward as you try to find the aerobic components that work best for you. Keep at it. Before long, you'll find the right mix of activities and fall into a rhythm. Here are some tips to help you get the hang of it and to maximize the benefits of your CR workouts.

Set a timer. CR training works best when you get as close to 2½ minutes of aerobic activity between sets as possible. But it can be a pain in the butt to keep checking the clock and trying to re-

member when you started. Keep a stopwatch with your weights and reset it between sets. Another great idea is to set an egg timer. That way, you don't have to fret about time at all. Just enjoy your aerobics until the bell rings.

Find convenient cardio. You can do whatever cardio activity you like. But I would suggest activities that you can dive right into without a lot of setup. Some of my favorites include jumping rope, walking or jogging on a treadmill, stationary cycling, stepping up and down on a step, and performing snippets of exercise videos. Choose something that's convenient and fun to do. And you don't have to do the same cardio activity throughout the workout. Mix it up for variety.

Lift slowly. Strength-training exercises are most effective when performed slowly. That's true in CR training, too. But sometimes, women get so caught up in an aerobic mind-set during a CR routine that they jump into the strength-training component and start swinging the weights like they're trying out for the cheerleading squad. Always count 1-2-3 as you lift and 1-2-3 as you lower. It will remind you to take your time.

Aim for balance. Work your body as evenly as possible by balancing your strength-training exercises with your cardio activity. This will give you the best muscle-building workout without overdoing it. If your strength-training routine includes a lot of chest and back exercises, for instance, you might not want to jump on a rowing machine for all of your cardio. Likewise, if you're doing squats, lunges, and stepups, then dancing up and down off a step as your aerobic activity may be a bit of overkill.

Recover and rebuild. Like regular strength training, you shouldn't do CR training on consecutive days. Your muscles need at least 48 hours between workouts to repair themselves and get stronger. If you find yourself making a routine out of CR training, do it every other day. On most off days, do some light aerobic activity like walking, hiking, cycling, or swimming for 30 to 45 minutes to keep your energy levels high. And, of course, you can completely take off for a day.

cardioresistance training stats

Here's what you can expect from **45 minutes** of CR training.

Calories burned
350 to 400 (based on a 140-pound woman)

Muscles worked
All major muscles in your upper and lower body

Psychological benefits
You have the satisfaction of accomplishing the entire day's fitness goals in one session.

Hydrate. Last, but definitely not least, keep a water bottle nearby. Your working muscles are going to generate more heat than usual, especially since they won't be getting any downtime between sets. Try to drink 8 to 12 ounces during your CR workout session, more if you're exercising in a warm room or tend to sweat a lot. And remember that you should be keeping yourself hydrated all day long.

astanga yoga

Flexibility and grace at a heart-pounding pace

You probably wouldn't expect to see yoga in the cardio section of a fitness book, but astanga yoga (also called power yoga) is such a vigorous, calorie-burning exercise that it definitely merits a mention.

Yoga is a series of postures, called asanas, and breathing exercises developed more than 3,000 years ago. Yoga, which means to unite or yoke, was originally designed to connect the body and the spirit. In practical terms, it relaxes tight muscles and ligaments; reduces stress; and improves balance, flexibility, strength, and coordination. Even though yoga disciplines that are popular in the United States, like hatha yoga, have long been touted for all the healthy benefits they provide, they weren't useful for working up a sweat or kicking your body into bikini-ready shape.

Astanga yoga has changed that. This style of yoga uses many of the traditional postures to stretch and strengthen your muscles. Instead of having you pause between them, however, astanga yoga flows them together in a continuous series that raises your heart rate and challenges your heart and lungs as well as your muscles and mind. Speaking of muscles, this workout also helps you build *beautiful* muscles. Celebrities like Sting, Madonna, and Kareem Abdul-Jabbar credit rigorous yoga workouts for their sexy muscle tone and physiques.

Getting Started

Here's an aerobic activity you *don't* need proper footwear for. In fact, you can do it in your bare feet. If you do wear shoes—and that might be a good idea if you're just starting out and are a little wobbly on your feet since astanga yoga requires a fair amount of balance—look for a pair of light sports shoes with a very flexible sole. The shoe should bend easily between your hands.

For a good at-home workout, choose a room with high ceilings where you can reach overhead without hitting hanging lamps or fans. And if the floor isn't carpeted, invest in a yoga mat. You can buy one for about $20 at almost any discount department store. These mats are designed with nonskid backings so that they won't give way beneath your feet at inopportune times. Many are even machine washable, which is a big plus if you tend to sweat a lot.

Yoga is a perfect at-home workout, but if it's a brand-new activity for you, do yourself a favor and take one class a week and use a video for your at-home workouts. A few sessions with a certified instructor will give you a better understanding of how to approach yoga poses, so you'll be more confident when you're on your own. Check your local Y for classes.

There are myriad books that detail yoga asanas, but I highly recommend picking up a video and following that. Your workout will flow better and you'll be more likely to perform postures correctly if a "live" instructor is leading the way. Good tapes include Bryan Kest's *Power Yoga* series and Baron Baptiste's *Hot Yoga 1*. Aim for 2

between YOU&ME

I went into my first power yoga class feeling very cocky and thinking it would be a breeze because I'm strong and lift weights. Besides, I had taken basic yoga before. Ha! Ten minutes into the class, my muscles were quivering, my skin was flushed like I was on fire, and I was praying to make it through the moves without collapsing. Pleasantly humbled, I have a new appreciation for this discipline. If you love yoga but miss a good sweat, this is for you.

to 3 sessions a week, doing some light activity like walking on alternate days.

Tips and Techniques

Yoga is totally unlike any other exercise, so you're going to feel awkward the first few times, but in a fun, learning-new-things kind of way. Keep at it; before long, you'll be striking poses with confidence and strength. The following tips can help.

Modify at will. Yoga is all about expanding your body's natural flow, not forcing it into painful positions. If you can't perform a posture, do a modified version. All good instructors and videos will show alternate ways to perform asanas for people of all strength and flexibility levels. Everyone's body is different, so there's no shame in adapting the postures to suit your needs.

Stretch just so far. Yoga is a low-risk activity. When people do injure themselves, it's from overstretching. Remember that this isn't a competition. Just because one woman can wrap her arms around her calves and give them a hug doesn't mean you should feel obligated to try the same thing. Stretching farther than is comfortable can stress your connective tissues and actually make them weaker rather than stronger over time. Stop when you feel mild discomfort. And relax, flexibility will come.

astanga yoga stats

Here's what you get from a **50-minute** class.

Calories burned
318 (based on a 140-pound woman)

Muscles worked
You name it

Psychological benefits
You get huge stress relief and a feeling of mind-body connectedness. In addition, yoga stretches your muscles as you strengthen them, leaving them stronger and more flexible in one unique workout.

BRUSHING UP ON THE BASICS

Yoga is easier once you know some of the basic moves. Here are three simple poses that you'll return to again and again in yoga class. Learn these, and you'll feel more confident right from the start.

❏ **Downward dog.** Lying facedown on the floor with your palms at your armpits, press up onto your hands and feet. Press into the floor with your hands and feet, straightening your arms and legs and raising your hips toward the ceiling so that your body forms an inverted V. Your heels will naturally come off the floor, and your knees may bend if your hamstrings are tight. As you relax into the pose, try to press your sit bones (the two bones deep in your glutes that you sit on) toward the ceiling and your heels to the floor. Hold for four or five breaths.

❏ **Upward dog, or cobra.** Lie facedown with your palms on the floor just in front of your shoulders. Lift your chin off the floor and slowly straighten your arms, raising your upper body off the floor. Come up as far as is comfortable without overarching your back. For an easier variation, keep your forearms on the floor and rest on your elbows instead of your hands. Hold for four or five breaths.

❏ **The warrior.** From a standing position, take a giant step forward with your right leg, bending your right knee. Pivot your back heel inward. Raise your chin and look slightly upward as you raise your arms up over your head, with your palms facing in. Hold for four breaths. Repeat with the other leg.

power walking

Blast fat with this quick-step approach

Thousands of doctors recommend it. Hundreds of studies extol its benefits. It's simple. It's enjoyable. You can do it virtually anywhere. Yet when it comes to building muscle and burning fat, many women refuse to take walking seriously.

It's understandable. In our more-is-better culture, it's easy to turn up our noses at walking as something people do when they're not fit enough to jog or run. But when it's done right, walking can blast away fat as fast as jogging—maybe faster. Even better, walking is easier on your joints, since you hit the ground with less than half the force you do when you jog. As a result, you're less likely to have your fitness goals sidelined by soreness or injury.

The secret is shifting from the typical window-shopping stroll to a more athletic gait and pace. It takes a little practice, but the payoff is a lower-body makeover that'll definitely put some strut in your step.

Getting Started

This is a moderate-impact aerobic activity, so you *know* the first thing you have to do is get yourself some good shoes. Prevent sore, achy feet by wearing walking shoes that are light, roomy, and flexible. When you bend the shoe, it should yield easily at the ball of the foot. When it's on your foot, there should be a thumb's width of space from the end of your longest toe to the front of the shoe. If your shoes are too stiff or too tight, you'll be battling tingling toes and achy joints 20 minutes into the walk.

Next, you want to work on your pace. For optimum calorie burning, I recommend aiming to walk at about a 4½-mile per hour (mph) pace. Fitness scientists at Washington University in St. Louis have discovered that if you walk at this pace, you can burn almost as many calories (201 per 30 minutes, based on a 140-pound woman) as someone jogging at about the same speed (223 calories per 30 minutes) because you're using the same amount of energy to stay in motion. Of course 4½ mph is a fast walk; if you haven't been walking regularly, you shouldn't expect to hit that speed right out of the gate. Start at a slower pace and use the same fat-burning walking form to work up to 4½ mph.

To find your current pace, go to your local high school running track (it should measure ¼ mile) or take a drive and measure a mile around the neighborhood with your car's odometer. Then go out and walk the mile. If it takes you 20 minutes, that's 3 mph; 15 minutes is 4 mph; 13 minutes is 4½ mph, and 12 minutes is a highly athletic 5 mph. The brisker your pace, the more calories you will burn. But if all you can manage is a 20-minute mile, don't worry. Walk regularly, and within 3 weeks, your pace and endurance will increase.

Aim for 4 to 6 power walks a week. Beginners

power walking stats

Here's what you get from **45 minutes** of striding.

Calories burned
214 (4½-mile-per-hour pace, based on a 140-pound woman)

Muscles worked
Abdominals, hip flexors, quadriceps, hamstrings, glutes, and gastrocnemius

Psychological benefits
Walking clears your mind and washes away stress. Plus, you can feel great knowing that your walking routine strengthens your heart; lowers your blood pressure; and dramatically lowers your odds of developing diabetes, some cancers, and depression.

should strive to stride for 20 to 30 minutes. More experienced walkers can step it up to 45- or even 60-minute sessions (when time allows). As a rule of thumb, increase your workout time by 10 percent a week. So if you're currently walking 30 minutes a day, 4 days a week, then you should add only 12 minutes to your total weekly walking time the first week you increase. Remember that your workout time includes a few minutes to warm up and a few minutes to cool down and stretch.

Tips and Techniques

It's supereasy to walk off extra weight if you start walking the right way. Here's how to transform your everyday stroll into a fat-blasting, muscle-toning stride.

Roll heel, ball, toe. Tell most women to pick up the pace, and they will immediately lengthen their strides. But long strides are actually less efficient and more tiring than quick heel-ball-toe steps. To perform the proper quick-step stride, concentrate on landing on your heels, rolling through your instep, then propelling yourself with a push off your toes. You'll be surprised at how fast these little steps can be.

Hold your head high. While it's important to watch where you're going, you don't want your head to hang down toward your feet. Raise your chin up and look about 10 feet ahead of you. This will give you plenty of peripheral vision to see the sidewalk below yet still keep your neck and head in picture-perfect posture.

Swing your fists. Instead of letting your arms hang down loosely by your sides, bend your elbows 90 degrees, close your hands in relaxed fists, and swing them in an arc from your waist to your chest, keeping them close to your body. By swinging your arms, you'll walk faster, burn more calories, build upper-body strength, and keep your fingers from swelling the way they often do after you've walked for a while.

Zip up. For a stronger stride, suck your abdominal muscles in and up like you're zipping a snug pair of jeans. Contracting your abs not only helps tone your tummy, but also supports your spine so that you maintain proper posture while you walk.

Tighten your butt. Your glute muscles are the engine that puts power in your stride. Make these muscles work even better by keeping them active as you exercise. Hold your butt muscles taut and contracted as you walk by pretending to squeeze a dollar bill between them (it's silly, but it

works) as you walk. As a bonus, your glutes will get firmer faster.

Pretend you're late. If you're still not sure how fast you should be walking, here's a quick, measurement-free way to remember. Pick up your pace to the point where you're just about ready to break into a jog. That's about where you want to hover for most of your walk. Your pace should feel as it would if you were running late for an important appointment.

Add intervals. If you can't quite sustain the speedy pace you'd like, add intervals to your workouts; it's the fastest way to get quicker and fitter. Although the term sounds intimidating, *interval training* means nothing more than adding quick bursts of speed to your workout. Do this on just 2 nonconsecutive days a week (walk at your usual pace on the other days) and you'll burn megacalories as well as increase your walking speed. Here are a few 30-minute interval sessions to try. For all interval sessions, judge your exertion on a scale of 1 to 10, with 1 being standing still and 10 being on the verge of exhaustion.

❏ **Classic pyramid.** This simple interval session gradually builds in intensity to a peak, then eases back down.

Pace	Min	Exertion (1 to 10)
Warmup	5	5
Typical	5	6
Brisker than usual	4	7
Fastest possible	2	8
Brisker than usual	4	7
Typical	5	6
Cooldown	5	5

❏ **Peaks and valleys.** This workout combines big blasts of speed with slower recovery breaks.

Pace	Min	Exertion (1 to 10)
Warmup	5	5
Typical	3	6
Fastest possible	2	8
Typical	3	6
Fastest possible	2	8
Typical	3	6
Fastest possible	3	8
Typical	4	6
Cooldown	5	5

❏ **Crazy 8s.** This workout is a fun mishmash of moderate- to high-intensity intervals.

Pace	Min	Exertion (1 to 10)
Warmup	5	5
Brisker than usual	8	7
Typical	4	6
Brisker than usual	4	7
Fastest possible	2	8
Typical	2	6
Cooldown	5	5

Take it to the trails. Most towns and cities have walking paths, city parks, and local nature trails. Use them. Getting off the sidewalk and into green spaces is a great break for your mind and body. Plus, you burn more calories on soft, varying terrain. If you're not sure where to find them, check your local library or the Internet for information on walking paths in your area. Or just ask in your local sporting goods store. The clerks usually know the great places to exercise outside.

world-dance aerobics

A fat-blasting party mix

T he days of mindless bobbing up and down to high-speed disco remixes are over. A new generation of aerobic dance classes has swept the nation. Unlike the stilted grapevines and pom-pom girl moves of the old 1980s-style dance classes, these classes really rock.

Spin and whirl to Bahamian rhythms; shake your hips to Jamaican-style reggae; or jump and jive to hip-hop and funk. The selection is limitless. Some classes even serve up a whole-world party, melding together moves borrowed from African tribal, Cuban, Brazilian, and other high-energy ethnic dances. The music is hip and fresh. The choreography is new and exciting. And as a side benefit, you get to blast fat off your hips, butt, and thighs.

Here's more news worth dancing about. Many of these classes are available on videotape, so even if you're the shyest of wallflowers, you can feel free to shake and shimmy in the privacy of your own living room.

Getting Started

Although you could just throw on some music and dance on your own, you'll get a better workout and learn some new moves if you follow an instructor. To find a class in your area, pick up the phone book and call around. Some dance studios are open for aerobic dance classes in the evenings. YWCAs offer a variety of classes. And some gyms will allow you to pay for classes rather than having to pay a full membership fee.

If video workouts are your preference, head to your local sporting goods or discount chain store, or even the Internet, and check out the selection. Look for a video that is suited to your fitness level. If you have been very sedentary for the past year or are fairly overweight, start with a beginner's tape. Women who exercise a few times a week can start with intermediate-level tapes. The advanced tapes are best suited for longtime aerobic-dance enthusiasts. Also, be sure to check the workout time. Some tapes run as long as 75 minutes. If you have only 30 to 45 minutes to exercise, buy shorter videos that will give you a full workout, complete with warmup, cooldown, and stretching in that time frame.

Once you have a class or tape to dance to, you'll need some dancing shoes. And that doesn't mean stiletto heels, although I've seen women show up to classes in everything from boat shoes to bare feet. A supportive, well-cushioned pair of cross-training shoes will help absorb the impact as you step and kick. Even if you're dancing on a carpeted or matted floor, shoes are a good idea to provide ankle support and heel control.

Try to dance 4 days a week for 30 to 60 min-

world-dance aerobics stats

Here's what you get from **45 minutes** of moving to the music.

Calories burned
286 (based on a 140-pound woman)

Muscles worked
Quadriceps, hamstrings, glutes, hip flexors, abdominals, and depending on the dance, deltoids and back

Psychological benefits
The music and moves will lift your mood. You're guaranteed to leave smiling.

utes, depending on your fitness level and the amount of time you have available.

Tips and Techniques

Every dance class uses a different technique, so it usually takes a few sessions to fall into a rhythm and start really having fun. The following tips will help you get into the swing of things.

Grab a partner. It takes a fair amount of courage to step into an established aerobic dance class for the first time. No matter how old we get, "new kid" syndrome seems to tag along. Even though it doesn't take more than a couple of classes to become a regular, some women still find it easier to take a friend the first few times. The real benefit to having a buddy (provided she continues the class with you) is that you can kick each other in the butt on those days when one of you doesn't feel like working out.

Choose comfy clothes. When aerobic dance

first became all the rage, many women refused to try it simply because they didn't want to wear *those* clothes—"those" being the seemingly obligatory leotard and thong bodysuit. That unflattering uniform thankfully went the way of leg warmers. Today, you'll fit right in no matter what you wear. But for comfort, the best choice is a pair of bike shorts or tights, a sports bra, and a shirt made of synthetic material that will wick away moisture when you start to sweat.

Opt for the floor work. Many dance classes and videotapes offer a short session of toning exercises like abdominal crunches and leg lifts at the end of class. These allow you to focus on your trouble spots and build a little extra muscle. If you can spare the extra few minutes, you'll reap better results.

Ask for an entry-level lesson. The most difficult part of aerobic dance can be trying to follow in the steps of a fleet-footed instructor. The secret is in learning the core moves of a class because it then becomes a matter of simply putting

between YOU&ME

I've trained lots of women who absolutely love to dance. But they totally hate aerobics classes. And their partners won't go dancing with them. So they bitch . . . and eat. Maybe this describes you; if so, here's a better idea. Go take a dance class. Many community centers and dance studios offer truly fabulous classes in African, Latin, and other ethnic dances. You don't need a partner to join the group. And it still counts as exercise even if you're not in a gym.

the steps together in repetition. Many classes offer introductory sessions to help newcomers start out on the right foot. Ask your instructor if lessons are available. If you're using a videotape, watch it once or twice to get a feeling for the moves before you try to match the instructor step for step.

elliptical training

The latest home-fitness rage

Do you want a workout that combines the calorie-burning benefits of a treadmill with the lower-body toning of a stair stepper? Then step on up to an elliptical trainer. These versatile pieces of equipment are giving treadmills a run for their money as the most favored exercise machine in both homes and health clubs. And with good reason. There's no impact, so they're easy on the joints. They offer variable incline and resistance levels, so they're more versatile than a stair-stepping machine. And they get your heart pumping as well as, if not better than, any other exercise machine.

Elliptical trainers have two large foot pads that move along rails in an oval (or elliptical) pattern. The machine is programmable, so you can set it to a flat or very steep incline, or a varying combination of flats and hills to simulate real terrain. When the pads are at their lowest incline, the motion is similar to cross-country skiing. Increase the incline, and it feels more like jogging. Crank it all the way up, and it's like hiking uphill.

The real beauty is that elliptical-training workouts are much more intense than you perceive them to be. You know exactly how hard you're working on a treadmill, but moving at the same intensity on an elliptical trainer feels like you're just strolling along. This makes it ideal for women who usually avoid exertion. I've seen women who would never work out on gym equipment fall in love with and lose lots of weight on these machines.

Getting Started

You can do elliptical training either at the gym or in your home. If you choose to use the machines at a health club, first visit the club when you plan to work out and see how heavily used they are. Elliptical trainers are often the most popular machines in the place, and the waiting list can be long during prime hours, like after work, if the club doesn't have enough machines for the size of its membership. Many gyms will put a 30-minute time limit on their use during busy parts of the day to ensure that everyone gets a chance to use one. But you also can ask the staff when the elliptical trainers are most available. Coming in a half-hour earlier or later can make all the difference in the length of time you have to wait.

Should you fall head over heels for elliptical training, you can buy a home model. The biggest advantage is that you can use it while watching your favorite TV shows. Plus, studies show that women who have home-exercise equipment are more successful at losing weight and keeping it off than those who don't. The downside is that elliptical trainers aren't cheap. A study by the American Council on Exercise found a direct relationship between the price of home elliptical trainers and their levels of quality. When *Consumers Digest* magazine rated specific machines, here's what they found.

The best home machine (the Precor EFX) costs close to $3,000, but it has all the features of a club machine, such as programmable incline,

elliptical training stats

Here's what you get from **45 minutes** on the elliptical trainer.

Calories burned:
358 (moderate effort, based on a 140-pound woman)

Muscles worked:
Quadriceps, hamstrings, glutes, and gastrocnemius

Psychological benefits:
You can feel great about getting a high-intensity workout without feeling high-intensity discomfort.

speed, and resistance as well as a display of heart rate and calories burned, and it's just as sturdy.

For those on a budget, the better buy is the Vision Fitness X6200. It retails for about $1,200, provides smooth elliptical motion, offers a large variety of workout programs, and even folds down for better storage.

Aim to work out 4 days a week for 20 to 50 minutes, depending on your fitness level. As you become more fit and confident, you can start increasing the speed, incline, and resistance (how hard or easy it is to push the pedals around) levels to make your workout more challenging.

Tips and Techniques

Elliptical training is easy. Just push the pedals forward, and away you go. But with all of its options, elliptical training has more to offer than just spinning your feet in ovals. The following tips will help you get more from every ellipse.

Try it no-handed. Most machines come equipped with side rails that you can hold on to for balance. Go ahead and use them to steady yourself as you get started. But then let go and allow your arms to swing freely as they would if you were walking or jogging. You'll burn way more calories if you don't hold on, and you'll improve your balance, too. If your model has moving poles, by all means, use them—you'll burn more calories.

Cross-train. With all of its different settings, the elliptical trainer has the potential to keep both your body and your brain from getting bored. Make the most of the machine by using it to mimic different sports. Try setting the incline on high for uphill hiking on Monday; lower the ramp and increase the speed for cross-country skiing on Wednesday; set the incline level about midway to simulate jogging on Friday; then mix them all together in one workout on the weekend.

Wiggle your toes. Because there is almost no impact on your feet, you don't need special shoes for elliptical training. But that doesn't mean you should ignore your feet. Wear shoes that fit loosely and comfortably so that you have room to

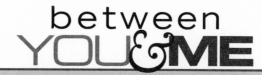

between
YOU&ME

I would rather endure back-to-back gynecological and dental visits than spend 45 minutes on most exercise machines. But when a knee injury forced me onto an elliptical trainer for rehab, I found that I actually liked it. The motion is very natural. And you can really get jamming and burn hundreds of calories without pounding on your joints or beating up your body. Just put on a pair of headphones and go.

wiggle your toes occasionally as you work out; otherwise, they can start to feel numb and tingly as you exert constant pressure on the pads with the balls of your feet.

Go easy on the reverse. Start stepping backward and you'll notice that you can actually mimic jogging in reverse on your trainer. It's kind of fun for variety, but it's not a good idea for an extended workout. That type of reverse motion is unnatural for your knee joints and can put too much strain on them over time. You're better off sticking to a forward motion.

swimming

Freestyle fat loss

There's no kinder, gentler place to work out than in the gravity-defying embrace of a pool of water. Swimming is easy on your joints, burns tons of calories, and makes you feel like a kid on summer vacation, all while giving you grown-up fitness and muscle tone.

Water is about 12 times as dense as air, so each stroke and kick through it is a mini strength-training exercise. When you swim, every muscle in your body is called into action as you push against the water's resistance. What's more, regular swimming can make you more flexible, something active women struggle with as they get older. Since you weigh only 10 to 15 percent of your land weight in the water, your arms and legs feel lighter and your range of motion increases as you move. Swimming also lengthens your body to its fullest potential, strengthening and stretching otherwise tight, shortened muscles.

The old myth that swimming doesn't burn off fat because your heart doesn't work as hard and your body hangs on to your excess "insulation" in the cool water is just that—an old myth. True, your working heart rate can be reduced by as many as 17 beats—or by 10 to 15 percent of your normal working rate on land. But that's because the force of the water actually assists your circulation in helping your heart do its job, and your body temperature is lower in the water, which automatically lowers your heart rate.

But that doesn't mean you're not getting a workout. Your lungs actually work harder against the pressure of the water, and your muscles put in overtime keeping you afloat. As a result, you're burning as many calories and conditioning your heart just as well as you would if you were doing most dryland exercises. Your lungs are getting an even better workout.

Getting Started

The first thing you need is a place to swim. For most women, the easiest solution is the local YWCA. For a minimal membership fee, most health clubs will allow you access to their pools. And general lap-swimming times are plentiful.

You'll also need a suit. This is the point where many women say, "Thanks, but no thanks." Relax; we're not talking about a flesh-flashing, butt-baring bikini. We're talking about an athletic, supportive swimsuit. You can even find boy-cut styles that look like shorts. Still feeling body-conscious? One trip to the pool will cure you. You won't see a bunch of bathing beauties; you'll see adult women who look just like you, who are there to get in some laps and get on with their lives.

In addition to a swimsuit, you'll need some other accessories.

Goggles. Because they're cheap and they save your eyes from the irritating effects of chlorine, swimming goggles are a must. You'll also see better while you're doing your laps.

Swim cap. Although it's not a necessity (though some public pools request it), a swimming cap is a definite nicety. If your hair is long, a cap will keep it from tangling. No matter what the

swimming stats

Here's what you can expect from **30 minutes** of a water workout.

Calories burned
255 (based on a 140-pound woman)

Muscles worked
Trapezius, rhomboids, pectorals, deltoids, glutes, and hip flexors

Psychological benefits
Cutting through the water is sensual, stress relieving, and a welcome silencing of the usual workday noise.

length, it'll protect your tresses from the chemicals in the water, which can dry or discolor hair. It's a good idea to look for a silicone cap. It won't pull your hair like a plain rubber one would.

The usuals. Don't forget a towel for drying off and a water bottle for keeping yourself hydrated (yes, you can get dehydrated in the water).

If swimming becomes your sport, aim to get to the pool at least 3 days a week. Beginners should try to swim 4 to 6 laps in a 25-yard pool. More experienced swimmers can float into the 8- to 10-lap range. And the female fishes in the crowd can shoot for 20 laps.

Tips and Techniques

Swimming used to be the sport that kept me out of triathlons because I sank like a stone and struggled just to stay afloat. One day, I got a few pointers from a pro, and my life has never been the same. By using the right technique, you'll go faster, feel lighter, swim more efficiently, and have more fun.

Roll like an otter. The more efficient your stroke, the longer you'll be able to swim. The secret is reducing your number of strokes while making maximum progress with every pull. Learn from the aquatic animals, and roll through the water. Contrary to appearances, swimming is not about twirling your arms and kicking your legs as fast and hard as you can. In reality, your power comes from your hips. As you move through the water, instead of just turning your head for air, roll your whole body, keeping your head in line with your spine, so that your mouth comes out of the water. Breathe, then roll back to the other side with the next stroke.

Streamline yourself. Your head should be mostly down, with the top of your forehead leading the way. This position helps keep your hips up and is less fatiguing to your neck than holding your head high and looking ahead.

Stay to the right. If you swim during prime hours, like morning and evening, there's a good chance that you'll have to share a lane with other people. Swim on the right-hand side of the lane, just like you would drive. If someone behind you is swimming faster and making you nervous, stop at the end of the lane and let her through.

Rinse before and after. Pool chemicals can leave your skin as dry as the Sahara. Avoid this ir-

ritation by rinsing off in the facility's shower right before you get in the pool and then soaping up with a moisturizing cleanser and applying a body lotion after you're done. If you're afraid that chlorine will turn your hair to straw, use a chlorine-removing shampoo such as Nexxus Clarifying Shampoo after every swim.

Switch strokes. Most swimmers do their laps freestyle, because that's the classic swimming stroke we learn as kids and it's the easiest to pick up. But you can work your muscles in new ways and improve your overall conditioning by playing around with a variety of strokes. Flip over and try the backstroke for a few laps. Learn the breaststroke or sidestroke. Your body will appreciate the new movements, and you'll be less likely to get bored.

gardening
and landscaping

A fitness activity you'll really dig

So you think that gardening isn't "real" exercise. Consider this: In a study of more than 3,300 women, researchers found that those who gardened at least once a week had stronger bones than those who were sedentary and those who participated in activities like jogging, walking, or aerobics.

And that's just one benefit you can reap from this nontraditional exercise. Gardening has been found to lower blood pressure, improve mood, build strength, and alleviate stress. As if that weren't enough, you can burn hundreds of calories as you dig, plant, and rake away, especially since gardening is easy on your body and there's usually lots to do. Women can easily spend a few hours tending the yard without thinking of it as exercise.

If you need more proof, take it from the fitness researchers at the Cooper Institute for Aerobics Research in Dallas. In a study that turned traditional exercise assumptions on their heads, scientists there found that sedentary, overweight men and women who did 30 minutes of nontraditional exercise like gardening and housework every day had the same improvements in fitness, blood pressure, and body fat at the end of 2 years as those who went to the gym for vigorous exercise 20 to 60 minutes, 5 days a week. If that's not enough reason to sow some of those wild seeds, I don't know what is.

Getting Started

There are two things you absolutely need before you can start gardening and landscaping: a yard and a love for yard work. If you file digging and weeding under "chores," I'm not going to tell you to start mulching for exercise. This kind of exercise is for earthy women who would much rather rake than run.

For those who are willing and able, the only other necessity is some tools. Although every job is unique, the basics are much the same. You'll need a few implements for digging, a pair of gardening gloves, a rake, some cutting or pruning tools, and a mower for the lawn. When purchasing tools, keep the following two guidelines in mind.

Go for hand tools. Since you're in this at least partially for fitness, choose tools that are human powered over those that run on outside energy. Buy a rake rather than a leaf blower. Edge your beds by hand rather than using a power edger. You'll also appreciate the silence of doing these tasks by hand rather than with noisy machines.

Comfort rules. Look for garden tools with ergonomically designed handles. You should be able to hold and handle them comfortably and without straining yourself. A pair of inexpensive gardening gloves with rubber nubs will prevent blisters and nail breakage.

And remember, gardening is literally an organic process. It takes the right amount of water, sunshine, seeds, and TLC to make plants grow. Don't feel bad if your strawberries are small or if

gardening and landscaping stats

Here's what you can expect from **60 minutes** of gardening.

Calories burned
318 (based on a 140-pound woman)

Muscles worked
All major muscles in the upper and lower body

Psychological benefits
You get a soul-satisfying workout that can put rich, beautiful food and flowers on your table.

your tomatoes freeze. It's a lesson learned in your labor of love. If you are a true novice, reading a general gardening book is probably a good idea.

For the best fitness benefits, try to do yard work at least 4 days a week for 30 to 60 minutes.

Tips and Techniques

Playing in the dirt can be a fun way to shape up and get stronger. These "fitness-gardening" tips will help you reap the maximum body benefits.

Take a lap around the yard. Hoeing and planting can be pretty strenuous. Avoid pulling a muscle while yanking stubborn weeds by warming up your body before digging in. Take a stroll around the yard, gather the tools you'll need, and stretch a little. When you're a little warmed up, start the job at hand.

Split your "workouts." Gardening is a total-body workout; some jobs demand more upper-body muscles and some jobs challenge your lower body. To use your muscles evenly without wearing any out, try to split your jobs according to the muscle groups they target. If you rake, hoe, and pull weeds (mostly upper-body work) on Monday, do chores like digging beds and mulching (mostly lower-body work) on Tuesday. That way, you always give your tired muscles some rest.

Watch your back. Shoveling, lifting, and planting will definitely strengthen your back muscles and improve your posture. But it's also important to use proper posture *while* you garden to avoid straining those essential muscles. The following tips from the American Council on Exercise can help.

❐ Let your legs help. You know to always use your legs, not your back, to lift heavy items like wheelbarrows of dirt and buckets of water. But remember to let those legs help do the work when doing small jobs like mulching and planting, too. It's better to do lots of squatting than constantly bending over.

❐ Turn, don't twist. When digging dirt, avoid twisting your back to toss the dirt aside. Instead, rotate your feet in the direction you want the dirt to go, and turn your entire body.

❐ Stand and stretch. The ground is pretty low, so reaching it means a lot of bending, kneeling, and crouching. Take stretch breaks

between YOU&ME

I live on fruits and vegetables, but gardening is not my bag—probably because my dad always had a list of garden chores waiting for us kids when we rolled out of bed each summer morning. But I will give gardening its due. I can't keep up in the yard with my dad (who is 30 years my senior) or my gardening gal pals, no matter how much I run, ride, and lift. It's the ultimate workout for women who hate to exercise.

every 20 to 30 minutes to give your back (and the rest of your body) a break. Simply stand straight and reach your arms overhead for 15 to 20 seconds. Your body won't feel as fatigued when you're done with your gardening.

Exercise your creativity. Gardening is one of the few exercises that also makes a fabulous creative outlet. Try your hand at arranging flower beds. Plant a variety of bright, beautiful vegetables. Try landscaping with river rocks and colorful pebbles. Then stand back and appreciate the fruits of your labor.

snowshoeing

The anti-winter weight-gain sport

t's easy to keep off extra pounds during the summer months. There are warm rays of sunshine, long days, and lots of outdoor activities. But when the temperature drops and the skies shade to gray, avoiding the winter fat insulation can become a major mission. Now, there's a cold-weather workout that can whip you into shape quicker than any of your favorite summer sports. It's snowshoeing—the fastest growing winter sport among women. It's easy, safe, and invigorating, and it incinerates calories like a coal furnace in February.

The excitement over this activity is due to the miracles of modern technology. Snowshoes used to be huge, unwieldy wooden paddles awkwardly strapped to your feet, forcing you to walk like you just got off a horse. But today's shoes, made of synthetic materials, are lightweight, flexible, and contoured. In short, if you can walk, you can snowshoe. It's not only easier than other winter sports like downhill and cross-country skiing, it's cheaper. You can rent shoes from some retail stores and ski shops for about $10 a day, or you can buy your own pair for less than $100. All you need is some snow, and you're off.

Getting Started

Like running or walking, the beauty of snowshoeing is its simplicity. All you need to get started are some shoes and a place to go.

You can snowshoe anywhere you would walk or hike. Although deep snow is the most fun, 8 inches of the white stuff is a sufficient base. Take a trip through parks, state and national forest roads, hiking trails, or wide-open fields. If you're really adventurous (and experienced), you can head into the backcountry. In northern climes, there are miles of trails designated specifically for shoeing. Call your area sporting goods outfitters or ski shops for the best places to go.

There's a surprisingly large array of snowshoe styles you can choose from. Which type is right for you depends on your size and weight as well as what you plan to do with them. If you're going to hike with a pack or a child on your back, you'll want a slightly larger shoe to support the additional weight. Otherwise, a medium-size shoe will do the trick. A rental outfitter or sporting goods salesperson can help direct you to the shoe style that is right for you.

Although they're not a necessity, a pair of ski poles can greatly add to your snowshoeing enjoyment. They improve your balance, especially on the uphills and downhills. Your legs won't fatigue as fast with your arms helping out. And as a bonus, trekking with poles burns more calories and builds the muscles in your upper body.

Since snowshoeing is arduous, aim for a time goal rather than a distance goal. Beginners should aim for 45-minute sessions and work up from there.

snowshoeing stats

Here's what you can expect from **60 minutes** out in the snow.

Calories burned
500+ (hundreds more if you're climbing hills, based on a 140-pound woman)

Muscles worked
Quadriceps, hamstrings, gastrocnemius, and glutes (plus your deltoids, pectorals, triceps, biceps, abs, and back muscles if you use ski poles)

Psychological benefits
Playing in the snow is a huge mood lifter on cold winter days. And the scenery is truly awesome.

Tips and Techniques

Snowshoeing is as easy as putting one foot in front of the other. But it's even easier—and more fun—with a few simple techniques. Here's how to get the most out of this cold-weather workout.

Layer up. It may be cold outside, but once you get moving, you won't believe how warm you'll feel inside. Smart snowshoers layer up like onions. Against your skin, wear a light moisture-wicking layer, like a synthetic-fabric T-shirt. Then add a cozy middle layer like fleece. Top it off with a weather-protective layer such as a warm windbreaker or a ski-type jacket or vest. As you get warmer, you can unzip or remove layers.

How much you need to bundle the rest of your body depends on the outside temperatures and how warm or cold you tend to be. Because it's winter, it's usually wise to wear a hat and gloves. Protect your feet with a good pair of warm, waterproof boots and winter socks.

Walk on the wide side. Modern snowshoes don't make you walk bowlegged like the wooden ones of old. But they *are* considerably larger than typical street shoes. To avoid tripping over your feet, walk with a slightly wider gait than you normally would.

Try the path most taken. Snowshoes make winter walking easier by letting you float on the surface of the snow instead of sinking in up to your hips. But they don't perform miracles. You'll still drop a few inches into the powder, especially in freshly fallen snow. Experienced shoers minimize how much they sink by taking trails that are already somewhat packed down by snowmobiles or cross-country skiers. If you must take the road less traveled, take along a buddy. The two of you can take turns leading the way and packing down the path.

Toe-kick when you climb. Snowshoes are equipped with metal spikes, called crampons, on the bottom. These help you maintain traction on slippery snow, especially when you're headed uphill. To climb on steep terrain, kick the toe of your boot into the hill. It'll grip the ground, and you can step up with ease.

Lean back to head down. For fast, fun, crashproof descents, keep your weight back over your heels and your knees slightly bent. You'll

between YOU&ME

My favorite thing about snowshoeing is that it lets you go anywhere your imagination wants to go. During a big snowfall, I'll wait until night falls, then call a few friends for a trek over our local mountain trails. The snow is so luminous that we don't even need lights. We shoe our way to the top, where we can see the snow falling on the city below. Hot chocolate never tastes better than when we get home after a snowshoe hike.

swoosh and slide down the hill like a skier, only you'll be much less likely to wipe out.

Fuel up. A few hours of snowshoeing can burn more than a day's worth of calories. If you're planning to be out for more than an hour, take a snack like dried fruit or an energy bar. Because snowshoeing is so easy, you don't realize how much energy you've burned until you're suddenly famished. And always take water. Even though you may not feel overheated or dehydrated, your body loses just as much moisture during cold-weather workouts as it does during warm-weather workouts. An insulated water backpack is ideal. Or you can carry a bottle in a pack close to your body so that it doesn't freeze.

rope jumping

Schoolgirl fun
for serious body toning

L ike millions of adults, you probably haven't picked up a jump rope since grade school. But if you're looking for a killer calorie burner (almost 200 calories in 15 minutes) that's simple enough to entertain kids on a playground, yet intense enough to help condition the world's most chiseled prizefighters, it could be time to grab a rope and brush up on some of those schoolyard rhymes.

Are you concerned that you're too uncoordinated or worried about your knees? Do you think you'll be bored? Wipe those common misconceptions from your head. With the right technique, jumping rope is easy to master, actually strengthens your joints, and is pretty cool to do. There are even group jumping classes such as FreeStyle JumpRoping and video workouts such as *Go Aerojump* by former boxer and astonishing rope jumper Michael Olajide Jr. that help make rope jumping fun and accessible no matter what your level of fitness or coordination. Or you can pick up a few pointers, hit play on your boom box, and jump-start your fitness right now.

Getting Started

The key piece of equipment is a good jump rope. For performance and quality, you can't beat a plastic beaded or segmented rope. This style of rope weighs about a half-pound, which is just enough weight to give it momentum as it swings around so you don't waste energy keeping the rope in motion. And unlike very light-weight materials like leather, cotton, or nylon, beaded ropes hold a nice wide arc and are less likely to tangle in midair, which means you're less likely to end up catching your feet and feeling frustrated. To test for proper rope fit, step on the center of the rope. The handles should come up to your chest.

Because rope jumping is a bouncy workout, you'll need good shoes and a snug sports bra. A quality pair of aerobic or cross-training shoes are the best choice because they have added support at the ball of your foot, which is where you land. Help your breasts stay put with an encapsulation sports bra, such as the Champion Action Shape Bra. Because this kind of bra holds each breast separately in a supportive cup, it's ideal for women with C-cup breasts or larger. And it's ideal for high-bounce aerobics such as rope jumping. You can find this kind of bra in any sporting goods store.

Once you start skipping, the key to success is taking your time. Even if you skipped from sunrise to sunset as a kid, it's going to take a few sessions to get back into a rhythm and to build your fitness. Rope jumping sends your heart rate skyward quickly, so don't be surprised if you have to stop after just 1 to 2 minutes the first time you try it. Just jog in place, catch your breath, and jump for another miniround when you're ready.

Aim to do your rope jumping 3 or 4 days a week. Beginners should try to complete one 5- to

rope jumping stats

Here's what you get from **30 minutes** of rope jumping.

Calories burned
318 (brisk pace, based on a 140-pound woman)

Muscles worked
Gastrocnemius, quadriceps, hamstrings, glutes, abdominals, forearms, and deltoids

Psychological benefits
It improves your agility, hand-to-eye coordination, and balance, so you'll feel more sure on your feet. Rope jumping is also second to none for building strong bones.

15-minute session. More experienced jumpers can shoot for 20 to 40 minutes. Remember that you can alternate jumping styles if one becomes boring. Or you can jump in intervals lasting a few minutes each, then take a break to jog in place or do calisthenics like ab crunches or chair dips, so that your total exercise time is about 30 minutes and you're jumping rope about two-thirds of that time.

Tips and Techniques

The great thing about rope jumping is that you don't need a lot of special gear or detailed instructions. With a quick lesson, good form, and a few ideas to keep it fresh, you'll be on your way to toning up and dropping pounds. The following tips will get you started.

Use good form. With good form, jumping is

easier and more enjoyable no matter what your fitness level. The components of the jump look like this.

❏ The twirl. Keep your elbows close to your body, your shoulders down, and your upper body steady. Holding your hands level with your hips, turn the rope with your forearms and wrists.

❏ The jump. Rope jumping is not a super high impact activity. You should jump only as high as is necessary for the rope to clear the space between your feet and the ground—generally not more than an inch. Keep your knees slightly bent throughout the exercise.

Do a ropeless warmup. Warm up with a few minutes of marching, walking, or calisthenics before you start skipping. Your muscles and joints will be more receptive to jumping, and your reflexes will be sharper.

Cushion your landing. The sidewalk was fine when you were a kid. But your grown-up hips and knees prefer a more cushioned landing surface. Hardwood floors, low carpeting, a thin exercise mat, and even blacktop are safer surfaces.

Keep the beat. Jumping rope to up-tempo music helps you find your rhythm and makes the exercise feel more like play. Turn up your favorite dance music and hop to the beat. With good music and a little imagination, rope jumping can be like free-form dancing.

Run, skip, jump. The classic jump rope move is a single two-footed hop per twirl. So it's

twirl, hop, twirl, hop. But you're not locked into this two-step jump. These moves not only add some variety, but also are easier on your body, so you can jump longer without needing a break.

❏ Single-foot hops. Alternate hopping with just one foot, then the other. Hop right then left for counts of one to three hops on a side.

❏ Heel kicks. With each jump, straighten one leg in front of you and touch down with your heel. Alternate back and forth.

❏ Rope jacks. Alternate landing with your feet in a wide or narrow stance, as you would during jumping jacks.

❏ Rope run. Lift your knees a little higher than you normally would and try jogging from foot to foot as you jump, so it looks like you're running through the rope.

CHAPTER 40

get off the scale

Meaningful ways to gauge your fitness

While you're getting in shape, it's natural to want to jump on the scale and check out your weight-loss progress. When you're strength training, however, that can be more deflating than motivating.

Muscle tissue takes up less space than fat, but it weighs considerably more. So while you drop inches and clothing sizes, your actual weight may move only a few pounds, depending on where you started. Larger women will lose more actual weight. Others may lose very little as they swap bumpy, bulky fat tissue for compact, curvy muscle fibers.

Breaking It Down

A body-composition measurement tells you what percent of your body is actually fat tissue and how much is lean muscle tissue. This is a much better indication of health and fitness than your total body weight is. For women, 17 to 24 percent body fat is excellent; 24 to 30 percent is normal; and above 30 percent is unhealthy.

Remember that you aren't gunning for zero percent. Your breasts are mostly fat, and you want those. Plus, you need at least 12 percent body fat to absorb essential nutrients and to keep your vital organs, like your liver and kidneys, working.

The two most common ways to measure body composition are the skin-fold test and bio-electrical impedance. The first method uses skin-fold calipers and is very accurate, especially if you have it done by a trained professional. But it can be pretty embarrassing to stand there while someone squishes your fat between these big pincers. The less embarrassing alternative is bioelectrical impedance. You step on a scalelike device (you can buy one for about $100; Tanita is a popular model) that sends an imperceptible electronic impulse through your body. Since electrical current travels at different speeds through fat and muscle tissues, the scale uses the signal to interpret how much of each you have. When used properly, these machines are pretty accurate. The downside is that they are extremely sensitive to changes in your hydration level. Exercise, alcohol, coffee, and general de-hydration can throw off your readings in a big way. So it's important to drink plenty of water, lay off the alcohol for 24 hours before the measurement is taken, skip your morning coffee, and not exercise for 6 hours before you step on the machine.

Or you can go an easier route and use circumference measurements to track yourself. Simply take a tape measure and measure around the widest part of your upper arm (you might need a friend to do this one for you), chest, waist,

between YOU & ME

Testing yourself is an excellent way to keep in touch with your fitness level throughout your life. But be sure to use the results as a general gauge for areas you want to improve, not as a way to slap another label on yourself. So if you can do only 5 pushups, you're not a wimp; you just have weak upper-body muscles. That's something you can and should change. By shooting to improve your scores, you'll have something to work toward. Even better, test your mate or a male friend along with yourself. Beat him in the flexibility test (women's hormones make them generally more flexible than men), be a good sport if he beats you at pushups (men have more upper-body muscle mass), and go head-to-head in the rest. That way, you'll both have something to work toward.

hips, thighs, and calves. Record those numbers, then measure yourself again in 8 weeks, after you've gone through your program.

Whatever method you use, remember that these are just numbers. If you're feeling great, looking fabulous, and fitting into your clothes better, don't get bummed out because your body fat percentage or thigh circumference isn't the number you wanted to see. Too often, women get a magic number in their heads (usually their weight in about seventh grade) that they won't let go of. Women's bodies change day to day and year to year. First and foremost, go by how you feel.

Behind the Numbers: Take Your Body for a Test-Drive

I recommend taking your body for a test-drive and seeing what it can do. For the best results, take these tests before you start your program. Then retest yourself at the end of 8 weeks. You'll be amazed at how much strength you've gained.

The Crunch Test

This exercise tests your trunk, or core muscles. Strong abs support your body so that everything from rock climbing to sitting at your desk feels easier. They also look supersexy peeking out from under a crop top.

❑ On a carpeted floor, place two parallel strips of masking tape about 3 inches apart. Put an egg timer nearby.

❑ Lie on your back with your knees bent, your feet flat on the floor, and your arms down at your sides. Position your body so that the tips of your fingers touch the first piece of tape.

❑ To a count of three (this ensures that you use your muscles, not momentum, to do the work), flatten your back and curl up your upper body far enough so that your fingers slide to the second piece of tape. Return to the starting position. That's one crunch.

❑ Set the timer or have someone time you for 1 minute.

❑ Do as many crunches as you can in 1 minute without stopping or breaking your rhythm.

HOW DID YOU DO?

Age	If You Did This Many Crunches . . .	Your Score Is
Under 35	50+	Excellent
	40–49	Good
	25–39	Fair
	10–24	Poor
35–44	40+	Excellent
	30–39	Good
	15–29	Fair
	6–14	Poor
45+	30+	Excellent
	15–29	Good
	10–14	Fair
	4–9	Poor

The Flamingo Stand

Lots of women think they're klutzy, when in fact their balance has just gone bad from years of disuse. The Perfectly Fit System will change all that. In the meantime, see where you stand.

❑ Stand on your strongest leg (usually the same side as your dominant hand).

❑ Raise the opposite leg so that your knee is out in front of you. Keep the knee of your supporting leg slightly bent.

❏ Keep your arms down by your sides and see how long you can balance.

❏ Close your eyes to make it extra tough.

If You Balanced . . .	Your Score Is
More than 30 seconds	Excellent
21–30 seconds	Good
11–20 seconds	Fair
10 or fewer	Poor

The Pushup Test

I'm convinced that upper-body strength is one of the keys to happiness. You can move your own furniture, paddle your own kayak, and carry your own backpack. And straight, sexy posture becomes second nature. Here's a quick way to check your upper-body strength.

❏ Get into a pushup position with your legs bent so that you're supporting your weight with your hands and knees. Your body should form a straight line from your head to your knees. (If you're already fairly strong, get up on your toes for a full pushup.)

❏ Keeping your back straight, lower your chest to about 3 inches (the size of a fist) off the floor. Push back up. That's one pushup.

❏ Set a timer or have someone time you and do as many pushups as you can in 1 minute. You can rest between reps if you need to, but only in the "up" position, not on the floor.

Age	If You Did This Many Pushups . . .	Your Score Is
20–29	36+	Excellent
	30–35	Good
	23–29	Fair
	17–22	Poor
30–39	31+	Excellent
	24–30	Good
	19–23	Fair
	11–18	Poor
40–49	24+	Excellent
	18–23	Good
	13–17	Fair
	6–12	Poor
50–59	21+	Excellent
	17–20	Good
	12–16	Fair
	6–11	Poor
60+	15+	Excellent
	12–14	Good
	5–11	Fair
	2–4	Poor

The Stair-Climb Test

Good anaerobic fitness means you can bound up stairs and hoof it up steep climbs without heaving for breath. Strength training will help make that happen. In the meantime, see where you stand.

❑ Walk up 30 to 40 steps (or walk up and run down a small flight of steps several times) without stopping. You can hold the handrail if you need to.

❑ Wait 60 seconds, then take your pulse for 10 seconds and multiply that number by six. (It's easiest to take your pulse by lightly placing two fingers on the side of your neck.)

HOW DID YOU DO?

If Your Pulse Was	Your Score Is
Less than 90	Excellent
90–100	Good
101–120	Fair
Above 120	Poor

The Toe-Touch Test

You want your body to look tight. But it should feel loose. You can accomplish that by stretching reg-ularly, especially after you lift. Here's how to check yourself.

❑ Stand with your feet shoulder-width apart.
❑ Keeping your legs straight (but not locking your knees), bend forward from your waist and reach toward the floor.
❑ Note how close your fingertips get to the ground.

HOW DID YOU DO?

If You Reached	Your Score Is
The floor (palms down)	Excellent
The floor (fingertips)	Great
Your toes	Good
Your ankles	Fair
Above your ankles	Poor

PART 5

PERFECTLY
FIT

the
attitude

priority number one

20 guilt-free tips for putting yourself first

When I ask strong, sexy women about doing after-work bike rides or morning runs, I am always shocked and appalled when they respond with, "My boyfriend/husband/lover won't let me." But then I realize that, more often than not, the directive is coming not from "above," but rather from within. Women are so hardwired to take care of family and friends first that they're not willing to risk even the slightest disapproval from loved ones to go out and do something for themselves. Many won't leave for even an hour, worrying that the household will be cast into upheaval if they do.

There are two major points that every woman needs to know. One: Making yourself a priority is the best thing you can do for your family, marriage, or relationship. Two: They can survive without you.

I know that it's easy to take a stand until you're heading out the door past a kitchenful of pitiful stares. I admit that it's not always a walk in the park for me, either. But over the years, I've armed myself with a whole list of reasons why we will all be best served if I go and work out for a while. Here for your empowerment are the top 20 benefits of making your fitness your number-one priority, gathered from the strongest, healthiest, happiest women I know.

1. Make yourself happy. Regular exercise helps make you happy. Literally hundreds of studies have found that to be true. Researchers at Harvard University found that 10 weeks of strength training actually reduced clinical depression symptoms more successfully than standard counseling did. Psychologists are increasingly prescribing exercise to treat mild to moderate depression as well as anxiety disorders and alcohol abuse. So the next time you're feeling guilty or facing frowns from the family on your way out the door, explain that exercising for 1 hour lifts your mood, leaves you feeling great, and makes you more fun to be around when you return.

2. Feel sexy. Women who feel good about their bodies have more sex than those who don't. And women who exercise regularly tend to be happier with their naked selves. What's even better is that vigorous exercise produces feel-good hormones called endorphins that make some women feel sexier after they work out. So jump on the treadmill, then jump on him. You'll both feel better about your sticking to your exercise schedule.

3. Play like a man. A typical golf game lasts 3 to 4 hours. And a typical guy doesn't wrack himself with guilt about going out to the greens for the afternoon. The same goes for softball, hoops, racquetball, or any other sports that men play. Embrace your active hobbies the same way he embraces his—with guilt-free enthusiasm. To reduce precious weekend time spent apart, try to coordinate your activities so that you're wrapping up at about the same time.

4. Get in touch with your thoughts. For many women, exercise time is thinking time. In fact, it's the *only* time many working moms get to be alone with their own thoughts. Let your loved ones know that you need this time to think—undisturbed. Without it, you could forget important things, like who you are.

5. Do it for a good cause. It's not that you aren't enough of a good cause, but some women feel less guilty about time spent running, walking, or cycling when they're also benefiting a favorite charity. Signing up for a run, walk, or ride to raise money for multiple sclerosis, diabetes, cancer, or AIDS makes you feel like you're benefiting others as well as yourself.

6. Go out and play, Mom. Your kids don't feel guilty when they want to go out and play; they get excited about it. Let them know that parents like playtime just as much as kids do. They won't always be happy about it, but it's a valuable lesson.

7. Avoid therapy. If left unchecked, stress can be your body's worst enemy. It raises blood pressure, tightens muscles, interrupts digestion, weakens your immune system, and throws a huge wet blanket on your libido. Active women are half as likely to develop depression and anxiety as their sedentary counterparts are. They sleep better at night and feel more energetic and relaxed during the day. And you can get a quality pair of running shoes for the price of one session with a shrink. Tell your family that instead of running to a therapist, you would rather just go and run off the stress of the day.

8. Have a goal. Write down your exercise or weight-loss goals and share them with your family. Tell them that you need their help and encouragement in reaching them. That includes pitching in around the house so that you have time to work out. Have a family celebration when you reach your goals.

9. Leave a love note. Most of all, your man wants to feel needed. Show him a little love by leaving a note telling him when you'll be home and that you're looking forward to seeing him when you return. The same is true for your kids. The smallest gestures make all the difference.

10. Make fitness dates. You can have fitness as well as social time with girlfriends, without taking tons of time for both. Instead of meeting for drinks and dinner, meet to go skating, jogging, or biking, or head to the gym together. You'll be able to chat and catch up on each other's lives, and you'll get your butts in shape as a bonus.

11. Make it a family affair. The family that sweats together stays together . . . or something like that. Although I have no studies to back it up, from the active marriages and families I've observed, I believe that's true. So instead of always working out without your sweetheart and kids, take them with you sometimes. Plan a day hike. Do a family run. Spend the day swimming and rafting on a lake. The more you do together, the more everyone will appreciate taking active time on their own, too.

12. Seek divine intervention. I talk to God while I run, often praying for guidance or just saying thanks for the good stuff in my life. It gives me a sense of peace, and I feel truly connected to my spiritual self as I fall into a zone of contentment and exertion. And I never feel selfish about forgoing mundane tasks like dishes and laundry for a long run when I know that I'm not just training my body but also feeding my soul.

13. Keep it in-house. I once trained a woman who had four children who were all under the age of 8. Complicating matters further, her husband was a traveling sales rep who drove long hours every day and came home too wiped out to hold down the fort in the evenings. When she said, "There's no way I'm getting out of this house to work out 5 days a week," I didn't question her. She bought some exercise equipment and strength trained and power walked around her kids' school and nap schedules. She never felt like she was straining the household by leaving for long stretches, but she was still able to get her body back into shape.

14. Generate conversation. Whether you run, swim, or take astanga yoga classes, working out gives you and your mate something to talk about. Consider your workouts time spent making you a healthier, happier, and more interesting person.

15. Make the most of what you have. You undoubtedly will have to make some sacrifices for your relationships, especially once you get married and start to multiply. But neither "wife" nor "mother" translates to "martyr." Although it's not something we tend to think about when we're young and still kicking, our lives here on Earth won't last forever. Whether you believe we go on to another place, come back here as turtles, or end up on another planet, this is it for now. Make the most of the body you have and live your life to the fullest, with no apologies necessary.

16. Job swap. Our foremothers fought long and hard to set us free from strict gender roles. Let's not disappoint them by forgoing exercise because we have to make dinner. You and your partner are in this thing together, so help each other out. If your favorite kickboxing class starts at 5:00 P.M., tell him you'll do the dishes and put the kids to bed if he takes care of helping with homework and getting dinner ready. Both you and your mate can spice up the household drudgery by throwing in sexual favor bonus points for overtime!

17. Weave it into the routine. We all function better when our lives have some routine. If you plot out a relatively consistent exercise routine, everyone around you will simply adapt to it and not expect you to be around during those times. That makes it more predictable and less stressful for all involved. If folks still have trouble remembering, post your schedule on a calendar where it can be seen by everyone.

18. Hang reminders on the wall. When I look around our house, I see countless reminders of why we make time for exercise. Pictures of us mountain biking in Oregon, running in Philadelphia, and kayaking in Maryland grace the walls and fill picture frames throughout the house. These smiling images of us in shape and having a blast inspire me to keep physical activity a high priority in my life, so that I can continue to be strong and fit enough to do the things I love. Even if you don't care about running up mountainsides, photographs of you looking your best at picnics and parties work just as well to help keep fitness in a top spot in your life.

That's the positive-reinforcement approach, which is my preference. I do know lots of women who prefer reminders of another kind. They have not-so-flattering photos showing what they look like when they don't make taking care of themselves a high priority. I have more than a few of these shots myself, and they're definitely powerful. Just don't beat yourself up with them.

19. Say thanks. Sure, you're entitled to work out whenever you darn well please. I'll be the first to tell you that. But like most of us, you probably have people who help you along, whether it's dropping you off at the gym, buying you a treadmill for your birthday, or just saying, "Hey, you look great," when you've lost weight or toned up. Be generous with your gratitude and say, "Thank you" to everybody. Say it often. When people feel appreciated, they are less likely to complain when your workout takes you away. And they're more likely to go out of their way to help you in the future.

20. Just do it. Okay, I saved the toughest tip for last. If you've left love notes, thanked everyone, counted your blessings, and hung pictures of your happiest, healthiest self, and you still feel wracked with guilt about walking out the door to work out, do it anyway. People are amazingly adaptable creatures. I guarantee that after the first few weeks of your new exercise regimen, the husband and kids won't blink an eye at your short absences. And you'll come to realize that they really can manage without you after all . . . at least for a little while.

everyday fitness

Use more calories, lose more fat

don't mean to sound like an old granny, but a lot has changed in 25 years. Automated teller machines have replaced bank lines, e-mail has replaced trips to the post office, and a few mouse clicks have wiped out many a trek to the mall. And that's just scratching the surface of our modern conveniences. We have hand-held electronic organizers, cell phones, remote-control channel changers and garage-door openers, fast food, packaged food, and moving sidewalks.

And every single one of those conveniences is making us fat. Fitness scientists estimate that we burn an average of 800 fewer calories a day than we did just 25 years ago. Let me put that in perspective. If today you started burning 800 fewer calories than you normally do, you would pack on an extra pound every 4½ days. This is why the national waistline keeps expanding despite the endless preaching that you hear about exercise.

Even our entertainment has become more passive. Home video games, the Internet, and digital video discs (DVDs) don't get your body moving like kickball with the kids. As a result, our kids are getting fatter, too. And it's not just a problem of aesthetics; it's a problem of heart disease, diabetes, cancer, and a host of other chronic conditions. It's also just a drag to have your body weighing you down and preventing you from enjoying life to the fullest.

Get a Move On

The more sedentary our society becomes, the more important it is that we not only exercise regularly, but also that we also get up off our butts and engage life in a more active way whenever we can.

Weight loss becomes much easier when you add a few simple tasks to your life such as mowing the lawn with a push mower or washing the car. A study from Johns Hopkins University in Baltimore showed that women who increased their levels of daily activity actually lost more weight after 1 year than exercisers who followed a structured regimen did. Try these tips to get your body moving more every day.

Skip dinner and a movie. The classic date is a two- or three-course dinner and a movie washed down with popcorn and a soft drink. It's a fun night and a relaxing time, and by all means should be included in your repertoire—but not every time you go out. Instead, get creative and treat your body to some active date-night fun for a change. Go to an amusement park. Hit the dance floor at a local nightspot. Take a tour of a museum. Or head to town for an evening of antiquing and window browsing.

Get crafty. Hobbies like painting, pottery, and decorating are fabulous ways to put more movement in your life. These aren't high-intensity activities, but you'll burn more calories by doing them than you would by sitting in front of the TV, and every little bit helps. You'll also feel a lot better when you're done and have accomplished something than you would after blowing another night in front of the tube.

Take a stand. If you're going to be on the phone for a while, work your legs while you work your jaws. Get up and walk around. When you're watching TV, get up at commercial breaks and throw a load of laundry into the washer or dryer. Get up and take stretch breaks during the day if you're working at a desk. Always look for the more active option even when you're not being active: Sit instead of lying down, stand instead of sitting, and pace instead of standing still.

Fidget a little. We all know women who eat chocolate candies by the handful yet never seem to gain an ounce. One reason for that might be their "spontaneous movement," according to researchers. Weight-loss scientists from the Mayo Clinic in Rochester, Minn., found that when they fed a small group of normal-weight men and women 1,000 extra calories a day—enough to pack on 2 pounds a week—the amount the subjects gained after 8 weeks varied from a measly 3 pounds to 16 pounds. Why the big difference? Some folks burn more calories even when they're not exercising because they fidget. Tapping your toes, changing positions, crossing and uncrossing your legs, stretching, and shifting in your seat can add up to hundreds of calories burned every day. Now there's an excuse not to sit still.

Dine in. You already know that you eat way fewer calories when you're at your own dinner table than when you're seated in front of an Italian menu. Staying in and cooking also burns more of those calories. Buying, chopping, and prepping the ingredients (as well as cleaning up afterward) use more muscles and calories than does telling a waiter that you would like the chef's special. The next time you're considering eating out, invite your friends over and make it a group exercise in your own kitchen instead.

25 WAYS TO BURN MORE THAN 150 CALORIES

The simplest activities can burn the most calories, especially if you make them part of your daily life. Here are 25 easy ways to burn 150 calories or more, based on **60 minutes** of activity for a 140-pound woman. And you'll find a comprehensive list of calorie-burners on page 275.

Activity	Calories Burned
Baking	159
Barbecuing	159
Cleaning the garage	255
Cleaning the house	159
Food prep, cooking, and table setting	159
Gardening	318
Grocery shopping	153
Ironing	153
Mowing the lawn (power push mower)	350
Office work (copying, filing)	153
Painting (interior)	191
Playing the piano	159

Activity	Calories Burned
Playing indoor games with kids	159
Playing tag with kids	318
Pottery-making	159
Pushing a baby stroller	159
Redecorating and moving furniture	382
Shooting pool	159
Shopping at the mall	153
Shoveling snow	382
Stretching	159
Vacuuming	159
Walking the dog	191
Washing the car	254
Washing the dishes	153

feeding a fit body

Fuel your muscles, nourish your soul, lose the fat

Aside from breathing, it's the most important thing we do. Aside from making love, it's the most sensual. Yet as natural and pleasurable as food consumption should be, no other activity has the power to make women more crazy, confused, or depressed than eating does.

Little wonder. When it comes to food, we're force-fed so much conflicting information that even registered dietitians are bewildered. Fat makes you fat. No, carbs make you fat. No, sugar makes you fat. One week, we're shoveling down rigatoni like it's manna from the gods, and the next we won't so much as glance at a noodle lest it go straight to our thighs. It's enough to make a weight-conscious woman say, "Forget it!"

And to that I say hallelujah! The truth is that there is no one evil food group, just as there is no single superior one. Instead, they all work in concert to feed our bodies and nourish our souls. Overweight happens because we lose sight of this essential role of food in modern society. No longer is food our reward—and our fuel—for a long day spent sowing crops or tending fields. It's become a popular form of entertainment. Stuffing our faces is a pleasant way to kill time as we sit in meetings or watch TV. We're filling up our tanks without working our engines. And that entertainment is what is making us fat.

Body in Balance

When you start living a Perfectly Fit lifestyle, food returns to its fundamental role as fuel. As you start moving your body the way it was meant to move, you'll also start wanting to feed it the way it was meant to be fed—with a wide array of healthful, fabulous foods. Sure, you'll still be able to indulge in some sweet and savory desserts. But those treats are just the finishing touches on a nutritionally rich diet. The following are the fundamental components of an active woman's eating plan.

Smart carbos. Without carbohydrates, your body can't exercise. They put glucose in your muscles, and glucose is what makes you go. Contrary to fad-diet dictums, carbs do not make you fat. High-calorie, low-fat, zero-nutrition junk food that also happens to be high in carbs (like fat-free cookies, cakes, and crackers) makes you fat. The secret to making carbs work for you is choosing smart carbs.

A smart carbo is one that has something to offer besides refined white flour and sugar. Whole grain breads and pastas, fruits, and vegetables are all excellent carbohydrate sources. These foods wrap their carbs in fiber and are filled with vitamins, minerals, and other healthful phytochemicals. When dietitians recommend eating 50 percent of your daily diet from carbs, these are the foods they would like you to eat. The carbs to skimp on are white bagels and breads, pretzels,

refined-flour foods like cake and cookies, and sugary stuff like colas.

Powerful protein. Protein is a celebrity food and is touted for its fat-shedding prowess. But the fact is that diets that are high in protein promote weight loss simply because they tend to be low in calories and usually cause some fluid loss, not because protein has any magical slimming effect. Your body really needs protein for building and repairing your muscles. About 70 grams a day, or 15 to 20 percent of your diet, does the job for most active women. The easiest way to get the protein you need is by putting a little on your plate with every meal. That will give you the two to three servings a day you need.

Like carbs, not all proteins are created equally. The best sources are those that are low in artery-clogging saturated fat but rich in other nutrients and heart-healthy fats. Topping that list is fish. Studies show that women who eat fish—that includes tuna in a can (20 grams of protein in 3 ounces)—two or three times a week not only lower their risk for all kinds of diseases, like heart attack, stroke, depression, and cancer, but also tend to be leaner. Other potent protein foods include soy foods like tofu, low-fat dairy foods, beans, and lean meats. Go easy on full-fat dairy products, hamburgers, and fatty meats.

As a bonus for adding a little healthy protein to your meals, you'll feel fuller longer. Studies show that protein increases satiety, or how full you feel after a meal, so you end up eating less yet still feeling satisfied all day long.

Friendly fats. Say it loud and proud—fat is no longer the enemy. Yes, gram for gram, fat still packs twice as many calories as either protein or carbohydrates, so a little goes a long way. And you should still go easy on the animal fats as well as the trans fats in crackers and baked desserts because of their artery-clogging potential. But a touch of fat in your food helps it digest more slowly, so you eat less, feel full, and leave the table satisfied. What's more, there are some friendly fats that can actually help lower your risk of heart disease, cancer, asthma, diabetes, and even Alzheimer's disease. For most healthy, active women, the idea is not so much to cut or eliminate fat from their diets, but rather to swap fats.

The fats to focus on are omega-3 fats and monounsaturated fats. Research indicates that omega-3's not only fight disease but also seem to

A DAY IN THE LIFE OF A PERFECTLY FIT WOMAN

How many calories you need each day depends on how much you weigh, how active you are, and whether you want to lose or just maintain weight. But generally speaking, a moderately active 140-pound woman who does some exercise every day needs 1,500 to 2,000 calories a day from a wide variety of healthful foods. Here's a snapshot of what 1 day's menu might look like. (Remember to drink that water all day long!)

Breakfast
1½ cups cereal with ½ cup milk
1 cup strawberries
1 cup orange juice

Snack
8 ounces low-fat fruit yogurt

Lunch
Turkey sandwich on whole wheat bread with mustard, lettuce, and tomato
½ cup minestrone soup
2 chocolate kisses
Diet soda

Snack
Handful of baby carrots and 2 whole wheat crackers

Dinner
3 ounces salmon and steamed veggies over 1 cup brown rice
Spinach and sweet pepper salad
Iced tea

Snack
Warm spiced milk and 2 gingersnaps

lessen the pain from menstrual cramps. You'll find these fats in cold-water fish like tuna and salmon. Eating fish twice a week will keep your cells stocked with this superhealthful fatty acid. Monounsaturated fats are one of the heart-healthy components of the much celebrated Mediterranean diet, and there is also evidence that they may help fight breast cancer. You can get the monounsaturated fats you need by cooking with olive oil and adding small amounts of nuts and avocado to salads and side dishes.

Fiber-rich plants. If you want to speed up your weight loss without feeling any hunger pangs, fiber is the answer. Fiber actually eliminates some of the calories you eat, sweeping them through your digestive system so fast that they don't have a chance to settle on your hips. It may not be the sexiest concept, but it works like a dream. Consider this: If you double your daily fiber intake from the average 14 grams to about 30 grams, you'll absorb almost 120 fewer calories a day. That adds up to about 13 pounds in 1 year. Because it slows digestion, fiber also helps you feel fuller on less food. That's important because so much of our food today is high in refined carbs and sugar while being low in fiber, so we take in tons of calories without ever feeling satisfied.

Fiber is abundant in fruits, vegetables, and whole grain foods. Aside from assisting with weight loss, it also lowers cholesterol and keeps your blood sugar and energy levels even. The one dietary tip that women rave about more than any other is increasing their fiber. Without exception, they feel better and lose weight. For the most benefit, aim to eat 25 to 35 grams of fiber a day. Here are a few examples of fiber-rich foods to get you started.

Food	Fiber (g)
1 cup barley	13
½ cup General Mills Fiber One cereal	13
1 cup raspberries	8.4
1 cup Kellogg's Raisin Bran cereal	8.2
½ cup navy beans	8
1 cup whole wheat spaghetti	6.3
1 baked potato (with skin)	4.8
½ cup frozen peas	4.4

Calcium. Every woman needs calcium to keep her bones from turning to Swiss cheese. Your bones are living tissue, and they need 1,000 to 1,200 milligrams of calcium every day to rebuild, especially when you're exercising. Calcium can also help you lose weight, fight PMS, prevent certain cancers, and keep your blood pressure in check.

Although more research is needed, scientists are just beginning to unravel the wonders of this bone-building mineral. During a 2-year study, researchers from Purdue University in West Lafayette, Indiana, found that women who consumed about 1,000 milligrams of calcium (the amount in about three glasses of milk) as part of a normal 1,900-calorie diet lost body fat and about 7 pounds overall compared to women eating the same number of calories but skimping on calcium. The scientists think that diets that are higher in calcium suppress a hormone that affects how fat is synthesized and stored in the body.

Are menstrual cramps putting a crimp in your

exercise program? Calcium may put the kibosh on that as well. Researchers have found that women getting 1,200 milligrams of calcium every day for 3 months cut the severity of their menstrual cramps as well as other monthly miseries, such as bloating and mood swings, in half. Plus, high-calcium diets have been linked to a reduction in colon cancer and may lower blood pressure. Milk is definitely one of the best sources since you can get 300 milligrams in just 1 cup, but yogurt and fortified orange juice are just as good. And don't feel bad for using the low-fat versions of dairy foods rather than the somewhat tasteless nonfat varieties. A little milk fat is actually good for you because it contains linoleic acid, which, according to research, may be useful in reducing the risk of breast cancer in women.

Strawberries and spinach. You're probably tired of hearing that you need to eat plenty of fruits and vegetables. It's not original advice, I know, but it remains the best out there. The list of benefits from these gorgeous foods grows longer each year. Women who center their diets around fruits and vegetables are less likely to develop heart disease, cancer, memory loss, vision loss, diabetes, and digestive diseases. And if health claims aren't sexy enough to get your attention: You *cannot get fat* on fruits and vegetables. These foods give you the opportunity to stock your refrigerator and eat all day long without worrying about your weight. The government would like us to aim for 5 servings a day, but that is the barebones minimum. For the healthiest, slimmest active body, shoot for 10 servings. It's not as hard as it sounds. One large banana counts as 2 servings, as does half of a cantaloupe. A large salad can

ABOUT ENERGY BARS AND DRINKS

Unless you're going to be exercising for longer than an hour, forget about fancy energy bars and beverages. These foods are specially formulated to provide quick, easily digestible energy during distance runs, long bike rides, and other endurance events. But many of them pack more than 200 calories per bar. Eating that would be counterproductive—kind of like having a candy bar before working out. A little snack in the hour before you exercise is fine if you're feeling hungry. But stick with a small banana or a few crackers, and save the energy bars for endurance events.

The same holds true for sports drinks, which have additional calories and sugar. Those brightly colored, salty-sweet beverages were created to replenish the sodium and potassium levels of 230-pound bucket-sweating linebackers playing in the heat on a football field. Unless you're exercising intensely for 60 minutes or longer, plain water is all you need to stay hydrated.

hold as many as 4 servings. Once you realize how vibrant, alive, and trim you feel on a plant-based diet, burgers won't look so good anymore.

Body rain. Dehydration wrecks your ability to exercise and makes you look and feel frazzled and haggard, as it leads to constipation, headaches, fatigue, and poor skin and muscle tone. Because bottled water is available from most street vendors, convenience stores, and soda machines, there's no excuse not to shower your insides with the 2 quarts of water your hardworking body needs each day. And if you don't like it plain, there is almost no limit to the flavors you can buy.

Proper hydration is especially important if you want to lose weight. Water helps your body metabolize stored fat. Research shows that a decrease in water intake will cause fat deposits to increase, while an increase in water drinking may actually reduce fat deposits.

Snack baggies. Fit women routinely snack two or three times a day. Stuff your briefcase and your snack drawers with baggies of air-popped popcorn, baby carrots, sliced apples, raisins, dried apricots, whole wheat crackers, and other finger foods. When you're exercising, it's natural to be hungry every couple of hours. By eating a healthy snack between meals, you keep your energy level high, feed your recovering muscles, and prevent stuffing yourself at meal times. Some studies show that your body also uses calories more efficiently when you spread them out rather than consume most of them in one end-of-the-day binge.

Chocolate. Fit women do not mistreat themselves with total deprivation; they realize that a little treat now and then is the way to prevent a big weight gain down the road. If you savor one or two chocolate kisses after lunch, you'll be less likely to spend the afternoon craving something sweet, then eating an entire pint of ice cream when you get home. Chocolate is not my thing, but peanut butter makes me melt. A little bit every day or so satisfies both my sweet tooth and my soul.

adventure vacations

Wake up your wild side with some reckless relaxation

The next time you desperately need to get away, don't just go somewhere, go out and do something. Face it, lying on the beach is pretty lame after the first 15 minutes. You come home fairly rested and somewhat golden, but the experience is hardly life altering, and that vacation glow fades 5 minutes into your first day back behind the desk. That's why more women are opting for active adventure vacations—crazy, fun trips complete with llamas, fat tires, whitewater, and sky-scraping vistas that slap your routine in the face and bring you back to Earth a new and much improved woman.

I became turned on to active vacations when I started mountain biking. Burned out on traditional tourist trips filled with overpriced booze and cheap trinkets, I decided to take a different route on my next vacation. I would mountain bike through the high desert of New Mexico. After 5 days of reveling in ancient petroglyphs, painted sandscapes, and towering elk, I knew I'd never do a vacation the old way again. And neither should you. Sweating your way through the most beautiful places in the world leaves you with a glorious sense of accomplishment, childlike awe over the rugged wilderness, and jaw-dropping stories to share with your piña colada–sipping coworkers.

You can kayak with whales in the crystalline Sea of Cortez even if you've never put an oar into the water. Most outdoor travel companies offer beginner trips so that you can dogsled, mountain bike, snowshoe, or paddle without any previous experience. They show you the ropes, then away you go on an adventure à la *National Geographic*. And who knows? You just might fall in love with hiking, biking, or trekking; quit your job; and move closer to the backcountry. Or you'll just have the time of your life. Here are a few trips to try.

The Whole Enchilada

Flipping through travel brochures is like walking through an Italian bakery. Everything looks so scrumptious, you hate to limit yourself to just one treat. So don't; get greedy and go on a multisport vacation. These trips combine two or more activities into one action-packed adventure. In the summertime, you can try hiking, mountain biking, and rafting through the majestic Grand Tetons in Wyoming, for instance. If you're a snow bunny, kick it in British Columbia with a dogsledding and snowshoeing adventure. Three-day trips usually run $500 to $800. Six-day trips fall into the $1,000 to $1,200 range (more if you choose an exotic locale like Nepal).

Canyon-country exploration. Try hiking, mountain biking, whitewater rafting, and canyoneering in the fabulous red-rock wonderland of southeast Utah, including Moab, the mecca of mountain biking. Get real-life lessons in geology and ecology, and learn about the ancient Anasazi Indians along the way. Contact The World Outside at (800) 488-8483, or log on to their Web site at www.theworldoutside.com.

Maine mushing. Do some dogsledding and cross-country skiing through the hemlock forests of the Rangely Lake region in the Pine Tree State. You'll learn to mush while getting acquainted with the stunning frozen shoreline. If you're lucky, you'll also see some moose. Contact the Appalachian Mountain Club at (603) 466-2727.

Grand Teton riding and rafting. This majestic Wyoming mountain range is the perfect backdrop for horseback riding, hiking, biking, canoeing, and rafting. You're guaranteed to see the wilderness from every possible point of view. Contact Gorptravel at (877) 440-GORP, or log on to their Web site at www.gorptravel.com.

Trekking Lightly

You and your own two feet—the ultimate in simplicity. But easy as trekking may be, never underestimate where those great legs of yours can take you. Hiking trips abound for trekkers of every fitness level. The best part is that hikers are allowed in even the most remote protected wildlands, so you'll be privy to the most pristine wilderness when you use your own two feet.

Geysers galore. Trace tranquil footpaths through Yellowstone National Park's wonderful wilderness. You'll trek past canyons, waterfalls, hot springs, bubbling mud pits, and spewing geysers. And keep an eye out for some amazing wildlife: bison, moose, eagles, and elk as well as Yogi and friends abound. Contact The World Outside at (800) 488-8483, or log on to their Web site at www.theworldoutside.com.

Northern guiding lights. Nova Scotia is an oceanic wonderland. Trek through charming fishing villages, over rugged shoreline, and past the protective watch of a rich array of lighthouses. If you're lucky, you'll catch a glimpse of whales in the Bay of Fundy. Contact Backroads at (800) 462-2848, or log on to their Web site at www.backroads.com.

Dirt Camp and Wine Tours

Get on your bike and take the ultimate road trip on either the dirt or the pavement. Work out your killer quads on the slickrock mountains in Utah, or hammer down the untamed Pacific coastline. By touring on two wheels, you can see more terrain in less time.

Carolina dirt camp. "Girls love dirt." That's the mantra among women in the mountain biking community. And you can get all the dirt you can dish at mountain biking outings specially designed for women, by women. The trip through Tsali, North Carolina, fine-tunes your dirt-riding skills (no matter what your level) and shows you the wild side of the Great Smoky Mountains. Contact The World Outside at (800) 488-8483, or log on to their Web site at www.theworldoutside.com.

Napa Valley spinning and sipping. Spin your wheels through five valleys of world-famous vineyards and past larger-than-life redwoods and Pacific coast magnificence. As a bonus, you get a tall glass of burgundy when the day is done. Contact Backroads at (800) 462-2848, or log on to their Web site at www.backroads.com.

between YOU&ME

Many women who would love to try adventure travel hesitate to take the plunge because they fear that they're too clumsy, unfit, or _____ (fill in unflattering adjective here). Nothing could be further from the truth. Just because these trips are athletic in nature doesn't mean they're chock-full of hard-bodied Olympians. In fact, quite the opposite is true. Working women make up the vast majority of adventure travelers; they aren't superfit, they're just active. Like you. So drop the fears of inadequacy. Sign up for a trip today and start living out all the stuff you usually just see on TV or lust over in magazines.

Rock Your World

I am in awe of rock climbers, with their sinewy bodies hanging off the rock face, always determined to take the hard way up. You can learn this amazing skill through a number of outfitters. They supply the gear, the lessons, and the assurance that you'll be safe and sound as you head for the skies.

Needles and peaks. Going up? How about going 14,000 feet up? You will on this climbing trip to Crestone Peak and Crestone Needle in Colorado. You'll get lessons, pack horses, and support as you shoot for your first summit. This is an accomplishment you'll draw strength from for years to come. Contact Gorptravel at (877) 440-GORP, or log on to their Web site at www.gorptravel.com.

Adamant climbing. Thrill seekers should head to Banff, Canada (one of the thrill-seeking capitals of the world), for an unforgettable journey that blazes new trails up unnamed peaks. This mother of all climbing trips includes helicopter drop-offs, fully guided mountaineering, and lessons on using an ice axe. Contact Gorptravel at (877) 440-GORP, or log on to their Web site at www.gorptravel.com.

Sea Worthy

Sea kayaking always sounded intimidating to me, especially given my healthy respect for deep water and the large creatures that dwell there. But then I took a kayaking trip through the Cascades in Washington State. The boat was *much* more stable than a canoe as I soundlessly glided through the pristine emerald waters. Instantly hooked, I bought a kayak of my own as soon as I got home. Short of scuba diving, sea kayaking offers the closest view of orcas you'll ever get.

Virgin voyage. Paddling from shore to shore among the Virgin Islands is a perfect journey for beach-loving reformed sun worshippers. This tropical trip includes snorkeling, beach-combing, and camping under the stars. Plus, you'll learn more about the islands than just the price of a margarita. Contact Gorptravel at (877) 440-GORP, or log on to their Web site at www.gorptravel.com.

Glacial gliding. Traverse the stunning fjords in the Alaskan Tongass National Forest. Try to keep your jaw from falling into your lap as you paddle through iceberg-studded waters past 3,000-foot-high granite cliffs and towering waterfalls. Seeing whales and other marine mammals is almost a sure thing. Contact Alaska Discovery at (800) 586-1911, or log on to their Web site at akdiscovery.com.

Skill Seekers

There is no limit to the skills you can learn while chilling out in some scenic locale. Scattered throughout the United States are schools that offer classes in golfing, tennis, scuba diving, race car driving, surfing, snowboarding, fly fishing, basketball, running, horseback riding, sailing, rowing, and spelunking. Thanks to the Internet, these adult camps and classes are easier to find than ever: Search the name of your sport and "lessons" and see what comes up. Always check a few references before you pay out any cash. Then sign up and get schooled.

a fit attitude

Shape up your outlook on life

We wanted to have it all. And after years of fighting, we got it. The career, the family, the house, and the car are all ours. Now if they would all just get out of the way so we could have some time for ourselves!

Between commuting and caretaking, trying to squeeze in an hour of exercise on most days of the week can be maddening even if you really love it. Social outings, family obligations, and regular daily deadlines are always getting in the way. But smart women can and do work out around them; it just takes a little mental makeover. Women that I race with, work with, and train agree that a fit attitude is the first and most important step to a fit body. Once you get it all straight in your head, the rest will follow.

Working Woman's Workout Guide

I hate to be harsh, but "I don't have time" is no longer an excuse not to exercise. Everyone is busy. Everyone is really busy. We are *all* swamped. Women who make fitness a priority still have time to exercise. Yes, it's tough to fit it in, but the benefits are enormous: lower stress, a better body, increased enjoyment of life, and the freedom to be less selective about what you eat. If you take the time to create a strong, fit body, you'll be better at all of the things that are keeping you from exercising now. You'll be a better mother, lover, worker, and friend. If the president of the United States can make time to jog, so can you. Here are some tips for the working woman who can't manage to work out.

Rise up. Life pitches one surprise after another as the day wears on, and by 5:00 P.M., you can almost expect a curveball that will waylay your exercise plans. Research shows that for many women, the best time to make time for exercise (and stick with it) is early morning, while the world is just waking up. By the time you get to work, your workout is done and the day is yours.

Take a power lunch. Scientists have confirmed it. Sitting all day long is horrible for your back and worse for your waistline. Skip the lunch buffet and walk, run, or hit the gym during lunch. You'll return rejuvenated and ready to tackle the rest of the day. Just be sure to pack a lunch or grab some grub to eat at your desk when you're done.

Blow off daily stress. If you check out the health clubs at 5:30 P.M., you'll see that the post-work hours are among the most popular times to work out. Without a doubt, a vigorous 45-minute session blows off the stress of the day. With soccer games and dinner plans, this time of day can be a bit tougher to negotiate. But one or two evenings a week are all you need.

Work swing shift. So you and your husband both want to work out, but have no one to watch the kids? Take turns. Active couples with young children find that swing-shift workouts are often best. He jogs between 5:00 and 6:00 P.M., she gets on her bike when he comes home, and they spend the evening together. It's not a perfect arrangement, but it's a practical solution.

TGIS and S. Most workout plans give you Sunday as your day of rest. I say, take Sunday—and Saturday—and celebrate the weekend with some great workouts. Go hiking, biking, swimming, or skating. Just do something. You know you

want to work out 4 or 5 days a week, so here is your chance to seize 2 of those days without the time constraints of work.

Get Your Head in the Game

Not to lay any pressure on you, but every choice you make determines how successful you'll be at getting fit and feeling great. Making smart decisions starts with having the right mind-set. If you believe that you're a healthy, fit, active woman, you'll start acting like one. If you believe that you're lazy and undisciplined, you'll likely blow off your workouts and polish off boxes of cookies. The choice is yours. You *can* be the woman you want to be; you only have to get your head in the game.

Write it down and check it off. Treat your workout like you do any other important obligation. Write it on your calendar. List it with your "to-do" items. And check it off when it's done. It's an overstated tip, but it works. When you write it in ink, you're more likely to do it.

Pave the way. You know that there will be days when you try to talk yourself out of working out. Make the job hard for you to do. Lay out your workout clothes the night before. Write your workout schedule on your calendar. Tell your family your workout plans. The more firmly your path is set, the harder it is to veer from.

Count your small change. Contrary to what many women think, the big Thanksgiving-like indulgences aren't the ones that make us fat. The everyday decisions, like an extra slice of pizza or handful of chocolate candies here or a missed lunch walk there, eventually add up to lots of extra pounds. Don't deprive yourself, but be mindful of yourself. Are you really hungry, or do you just feel like eating? Is there something with fewer calories that would fit the bill? The more small decisions you make to eat healthfully and get moving, the fitter you'll be.

Get self-righteous. Only about one-third of Americans get even a minimal 30 minutes of accumulated activity—that means just walking around—every day. By working out regularly, you put yourself in a distinct minority of healthy, vigorous women. That's cool. Allow yourself to feel a little self-righteous now and then. A pat on the back can inspire you to keep it up.

Get Your Mate Involved

I'll admit that working out with your mate can be an exercise in frustration, especially if your fitness or skill levels are dramatically different. But it can also be extremely rewarding, which is why I encourage women (and men) to try to find at least one activity they can do as a couple. It not only makes the relationship stronger, but you'll also be more likely to keep at it. Researchers at Stanford University found that women and men who started fitness regimens with their spouses were more likely to work out regularly and less likely to drop out completely than those who started working out without their mates. The reason for that is what scientists call active intimacy. An activity is more fun when you're doing it with someone else. The support and camaraderie you can get from a mate pushes you past the usual plateaus and boredom points. Plus, couples who exercise together report having better sex—prob-

ably figuring, "Hey, we're sweaty already. . . ." Try these tips for a better couple session.

Take a hike. Low-competition sports like hiking are great for couples of varying ability. You're just out digging the scenery, getting some air, and trekking up the trail together.

Try tandem. In the if-you-can't-beat-'em-join-'em spirit is the tandem. There are bicycles as well as kayaks and canoes built for two. If one of you is a lot faster than the other, a tandem is a great way to ride or row together without anyone being left behind. As a bonus, they're *really* fast when you get going.

Hit the weight room. By weight training together, you can both do your own thing, only together. And it's fun to check each other out while you get pumped.

Mix and match. Couples who aren't evenly matched at any one sport but are both physically fit can exercise together without doing the same workout. I know couples in which one jogs while the other bikes. Or she skates while he runs. Or he snowshoes while she does cross-country skiing. Get creative, but get out.

The Games Girls Play

Your friends can be either your allies or your enemies on your quest for better fitness. It just depends on what kind of friends you have. If they're mostly commiseration buddies who help you drown your weight-loss woes in ice cream, don't be surprised if they're less than celebratory about your newfound fitness regimen. If you're casting off some slothful ways, you're forcing them to look at their own habits, and they may even feel like

between
YOU&ME

Life is a game of momentum. Once you get rolling in a certain direction, you pick up steam and usually continue along that course, gathering like-minded friends with similar habits. For many women, that means eating, hanging out, gaining unwanted pounds, and dieting constantly. Changing direction is overwhelming because they start thinking of all the stuff they'll no longer be able to do. "But I get pizza and nachos with my girlfriends every Thursday night. . . . My husband and I love getting ice cream on Sunday afternoons. . . ."

The trick is not to think that far into it. Just make one step in the right direction, like lifting 3 days a week, and the rest will fall in line. You'll feel a little sexier and stronger. You'll throw in an aerobics class a couple times a week. And before you know it, momentum has carried you in a healthier direction.

As a former nacho-loving smoker, I can tell you that this is true. And it's never too late to get rolling. One of my most treasured clients is a 57-year-old woman. "I'll never quit smoking," she told me. "You may surprise yourself," is all I said. "You may not want to smoke anymore once we start exercising." One year later, she quit smoking, re-upholstered her smoke-filled furniture, and repainted her entire house. She has her own set of weights and a treadmill, and she walks 5Ks with her daughter.

you're putting them down. Although I like to think we're all beyond this kind of petty behavior, I've seen enough women submitted to sarcastic digs to know that we're not past trying to jeopardize even a friend's progress. Here's how the women I know handle it.

Make it about you. Approaching the subject by saying, "These Friday chip-and-beer happy hours are making me fat!" will undoubtedly hurt feelings and raise hackles. Instead, just say, "I'm feeling a little burned out on the beer. I think I'll stick to seltzer tonight." It's subtle. It's graceful. And it works.

Gather some girl power. Your girlfriends may feel like getting fit, too, but they just don't know where to start. Share with them what you're doing and when you're doing it, and invite them to join you. You may be pleasantly surprised.

Stand unapologetically firm. It is astonishing how much energy other people can put into your eating and exercise habits, especially if they're not happy with their own. No doubt you will run into friends and family who will call you out and make you feel like Public Enemy Number One for not joining them for pepperoni pizza or Double Death by Cheesecake Surprise. If you're really not into it, stand politely firm. Don't apologize, and don't argue. They'll soon get tired of badgering and learn to let you be.

Spin off. Surround yourself with active people, and you're more likely to stay active yourself. If your current friends aren't encouraging your exercise efforts, find some new friends at the gym or in your neighborhood who will. You don't have to dump your old girlfriends, just spend a little more time with the ones who make you feel good about the new you. After all, that's what friends are for.

keeping the spirit alive

Where to find motivation when yours is MIA

Many women have the crazy notion that active folks bounce out of bed every morning, lace up their shoes, and cheerfully run 10 miles before half the world is awake. We never bury our heads in our pillows and whine about the weather, our workloads, or how we would really rather sleep for another 5 hours.

And that's simply not true. Yes, many of us *are* out riding, running, and lifting before most of the population has hit the snooze alarm. And yes, we do find ways to fit fitness into our daily routines. But it's not always so easy. The difference between women who exercise faithfully and those who wish they could, but never quite manage to, is that active women know where to find their motivation when their will to work out is down for the count.

Whether you're a self-starter or a slow starter, there are easy tactics to help you commit to fitness and stay motivated, even excited, about your exercise plan.

Follow your heart. You'll be 100 percent more likely to stay motivated to exercise if you truly love, or at least really like, what you're doing. Think about it. When you were a kid, if you hated kickball, you didn't play kickball. You did the stuff you really liked, whether it was swimming or riding your bike. The same is true today. If you try jogging or joining a gym just because you think you should or because that's what the rest of the women at work do, you'll quit inside of 6 months. Instead, gravitate toward the things that really interest you. Did you play sports in school? Join an adult league and enjoy the thrill of competition. Do you like to dance? Try a dance-based aerobics class. If you do what you love, you'll be more motivated to make the effort to exercise, and the fitness will naturally follow.

Donate your efforts. If you don't want to work out for yourself, do it for someone else. You name the cause, and there is a charity group that organizes runs, bikes, walks, or holds triathlons for it. Sign up to run for breast cancer. Do a walk-a-thon for diabetes. Spend a weekend cycling to raise money for multiple sclerosis. These events not only give you something definite to train for but also they give you the satisfaction of working hard to help others. Events are easy to find. Just search the Internet for the cause you would like to benefit. Then call or e-mail the charitable society or organization that works to raise money for research and resources. Common ones include the Leukemia and Lymphoma Society of America, the National Multiple Sclerosis Society, the Avon Breast Cancer Awareness Crusade, and AIDSRides USA. But you can find an activity for practically any worthy cause that interests you.

Make it a stress retreat. Any regular exerciser will tell you that one of the things she likes best about working out is how she feels when she's done. As I've mentioned time and again, exercise makes you feel happier and calmer; it also blows off stress better than any drug you can buy (legal or otherwise). For many women, their daily

exercise hour is the only time they have for themselves. Using your workout time to sort through the stuff that's on your mind is a great way to motivate yourself to get moving.

Keep a journal. Putting things in writing makes them real. That's especially true when it comes to working out, so put a journal or log book in your gym bag and record your workouts. Include information about what kind of aerobic exercise you did, for how long, and how you felt as well as what strength-training exercises you did, how heavy the weights were, and how many reps and sets you did. Along the way, you can include your weight, body composition, measurements, or other fitness benchmarks. Log books are motivating because you get to see your progress in ink as the weeks pass. And the log book itself becomes a visual cue to get off your butt and get moving.

Find fit friends. Do you think peer pressure ends at graduation? No way; your grown-up girlfriends are just as influential as those high school pals. Maybe more. If you tend to keep company with sedentary women who think that food is the highest form of entertainment, chances are good that you'll find yourself surrounded by fried cheese, doughnuts, and lots of excuses to ditch your Spinning session. Hook up with some fit coworkers or friends, and you'll find yourself immersed in peer pressure of a healthier kind. They'll invite you to the gym, out for a walk, to the park for some inline skating, and out and about wherever they go. Who knew motivation could be so cool?

Work toward something. We all want to feel healthy and look great. But even fitness fanatics can lose sight of why they're working out when they're out to just "stay in shape." Setting concrete goals to work toward makes it easier to stay on track and keep yourself motivated. And forget goals like "lose 10 pounds by summer." Those weight-related goals are never as satisfying as you hope. Better fitness goals are ones directly linked to your activity. If you like to run, sign up for a 5K race. If you just started strength training, set a goal to be able to complete a set of 10 pullups by the end of the year. Measurable, meaningful goals give purpose to your workouts and motivate you to keep going.

Set up a soundtrack. As any fitness instructor can tell you, music can make or break a workout. The wrong tunes drag a routine down, while strong, up-tempo rhythms that you love make you want to move—and keep moving. Skim through your CDs and record all of the songs that juice you up and make you feel like dancing. Then turn it on the next time you lift weights or get on the treadmill. The session will fly by faster and you'll work out harder. I've recorded a whole series of CDs to accompany my workouts, so I always have music to match my mood. On those days that I really don't feel like moving, I put on the music first; by the end of the first song, I'm raring to go.

Please do not strap on your headset and go running down the street, however. Women need to have their antennae up and working when they're out and about. And music pumping through your headphones drowns out important sounds like oncoming traffic and potential hazards like dogs and thugs.

between YOU&ME

I believe that the rewards of working out come from the workout itself. The toned muscles and the happy disposition are the really big payoffs. But I also believe that women should reward themselves for sticking with their exercise regimens. Go ahead and buy that sheath dress you would never have had the guts to wear before. Treat yourself to a few CDs. Take snowboarding lessons. You've earned it. Allowing yourself some material rewards definitely helps keep you going.

Shake it up. There is nothing like walking around the same 10 blocks at the same time every day to sap your will to exercise. Yes, it's easy and convenient to do the same workout routine, whether you're going 3 miles around the neighborhood or doing 30 minutes of program 5 on the elliptical trainer. But sooner or later, you'll fall into a rut, stop seeing results, and watch your progress—and your motivation—drop into the slumps. Stay off this slippery slope by shaking up your routine when it starts feeling so familiar that it's practically stale. Make a left where you usually turn right. Head to a nearby park for your walk. Get on a new kind of machine at the gym. If you're feeling bold, jump into a new class. Your muscles, your mind, and your motivation will thank you.

Try new stuff. Like exotic foods, you'll never know what exercises you'll love until you try them.

I remember when I first read about Spinning. As a competitive cyclist, I thought that a bunch of people riding stationary bikes together was the silliest exercise concept imaginable. Then I took a class and became almost annoyingly evangelical, preaching that everyone just had to try this. I even became certified to teach it. Keep your eyes and your mind open to new exercise trends, and make it a point to try them out. Learning new activities keeps boredom and waning motivation at bay and also introduces you to something you'll enjoy doing for a lifetime.

Dump it for a few days. Even if you love your job, you still need a vacation now and then, right? The same is true with exercise. You absolutely need to give yourself a break from your exercise routine now and then to remember what you love about it and to appreciate how good it makes you feel. Exercise vacations also help you feel less shackled to your routine. Take a long weekend to chill out at the beach, finish some home projects, or tackle a juicy novel. By the end of your break, you'll feel refreshed and ready to get back into exercise with renewed vigor.

calorie chart

You have to burn off more calories than you take in to make those favorite jeans fit again. That you know. But as easy as that sounds, it can be a tricky equation to master. Sure, your treadmill or the machines at the gym can give you a rough estimate, but once you go play outside or get off the equipment, how do you know if the energy you used equals 1 slice or half a small pie? To set the record straight, I don't think any woman should live her life according to how many calories she uses. But it is useful to have a rough idea, especially if you're trying to lose weight.

Here's a look at how much energy you burn during 1 hour of one of these 40 popular recreational activities. The numbers are based on a 140-pound woman. If you weigh more, you'll burn more; if you weigh less, you'll burn less. That's one place where life is a little bit fair.

Activity	Calories Burned
Aerobics (general)	414
Backpacking	445
Baking	159
Barbecuing	159
Basketball (casual, shooting hoops)	286
Bicycling (moderate)	509
Bowling	191
Canoeing	255
Cardio kickboxing	445
Cleaning the garage	255
Cleaning the house	159
Cross-country skiing	509

Activity	Calories Burned
Fishing	255
Food prep, cooking, and table setting	159
Gardening	318
Golfing with cart	223
Golfing (carrying clubs)	350
Grocery shopping	153
Hatha yoga	255
Hiking with daypack	382
Horseback riding	255
Ice skating	445
In-line skating (brisk)	445
Ironing	153

Activity	Calories Burned	Activity	Calories Burned
Jogging	445	Sledding	445
Kayaking in calm water	318	Snorkeling	318
Martial arts	636	Snowboarding	414
Mountain biking	541	Snowshoeing	509
Mowing the lawn (power push mower)	350	Soccer	445
Office work (copying, filing)	153	Softball	318
Painting (interior)	191	Stair-stepping machine	382
Playing the piano	159	Stationary bicycling	445
Playing indoor games with kids	159	Step aerobics	414
Playing tag with kids	318	Stretching	159
Pottery-making	159	Surfing (body or board)	191
Pushing a baby stroller	159	Swimming (freestyle)	509
Racquetball	445	Tai chi	255
Rebounding (trampoline exercise)	223	Tennis (casual)	445
Redecorating and moving furniture	382	Trail walking	318
Rock climbing (indoor and outdoor)	700	Vacuuming	159
Rope jumping	636	Volleyball (casual)	191
Rowing machine	445	Walking (casual)	286
Running (9-min mile)	700	Walking the dog	191
Scuba diving	445	Washing the car	254
Shooting pool	159	Washing the dishes	153
Shopping at the mall	153	Water aerobics	255
Shoveling snow	382	Waterskiing	382
Skiing (downhill)	382		

JOURNAL PAGE

Exercise	Muscles worked	Sets	Reps	Weight (lb)

JOURNAL PAGE

Exercise	Muscles worked	Sets	Reps	Weight (lb)

JOURNAL PAGE

Exercise	Muscles worked	Sets	Reps	Weight (lb)

index

Forearm extension, for toning forearms, 100, **100**
Forward and back kick, for toning lower body, 81, **81**, **174**
Four-direction neck stretch, for stretching neck, 155, **155**
Free weights, 34–37. *See also* Barbells; Dumbbells
French curl, for toning triceps, 94, **94**, **174**
Friends
  exercise with, 251
  motivation from, 271
  sharing fitness with, 268–69
Front arm raise, for toning shoulders, 97, **97**, **187**
Fruits, in eating plan, 260
Full-body exercises
  ball swing knee kick, 63, **63**, **183**
  benefits of, 43–44, 46–47
  challenge of, 44
  chop and twist, 50, **50**, **174**, **183**
  curl and half-squat, 59, **59**, **180**
  ditch digger, 58, **58**, **180**
  dumbbell squat and upward press, 54, **54**, **180**
  kneeling side chop, 51, **51**, **175**, **184**
  lift, curl, and reach, 65, **65**, **183**
  lunge row, 64, **64**, **184**
  muscles worked in, 47
  opposite arm and leg raise, 52, **52**, **176**
  results from, 48
  rising and setting sun, 56, **56**, **179**

safety with, 48
in self-designed program, 190
sprinter start, 60, **60**, **180**
squat and reach, 53, **53**, **179**
standing lunge and curl, 57, **57**, **179**
starting a routine, 47, 48
step and extend, 55, **55**, **184**
sumo squat arm raise, 61, **61**, **179**
synchronized kickback, 62, **62**, **180**
wood chop, 49, **49**, **173**
Functional fitness, 23–24, 46

G

Gardening and landscaping, 233–35
Gastrocnemius. *See* Calf exercises; Calf stretches
Gears, bicycling, 209
Giant V, for stretching groin, 165, **165**
Gloves
  bicycling, 208
  workout, 13
Goals
  exercise and weight-loss, 250–51
  motivation from, 271–72
Goggles, swimming, 231
Groin stretches
  butterfly, 165, **165**
  giant V, 165, **165**

H

Hamstring exercises
  lying leg curl, 116, **116**, **173**
  standing hamstring curl, 117, **117**, **175**
Hamstring stretches
  leg extension and pull, 164, **164**
  sit and reach, 164, **164**
Hand-to-foot ball curl, for toning abdominals, 130, **130**, **180**
Hand wraps, for workouts, 13
Happiness, from exercise, 250
Heart disease, preventing
  with aerobics, 9, 197
  with strength training, 9
Helmet, bicycling, 208
Hiking trips, 263–64
Hip stretches
  crossover leg pull, 161, **161**
  stair stretch, 161, **161**
Hook, in martial arts aerobics, 205
Hybrid bikes, 208

I

In and out, for toning abdominals, 129, **129**, **179**, **184**
Incline fly, for toning chest, 150, **150**, **176**
Incline press, for toning chest, 149, **149**, **175**
Injury prevention
  in astanga yoga, 219
  in running, 212–13

Menstrual cramps, calcium for preventing, 259–60
Mental acuity, from aerobic exercise, 196–97
Metabolism
   increased
      from aerobic exercise, 196
      from strength training, 6–7
   of muscle building, 201
Monster walk, for toning butt, 111, **111**, **188**
Motivation, for exercise, 270–73
Mountain bikes, 207–8
Multisport vacations, 263
Muscles
   boredom in, 200, 201
   identification of, **47**
   imbalances in, 4
   loss of, with aging, 7
   metabolism of, 201
   recovery of
      after cardioresistance training, 216
      after strength training, 18–19
   tone of, from strength training, 4
   weight of tissue in, 242
Music, motivation from, 272

N

Neck stretches
   four-direction neck stretch, 155, **155**
   side-to-side stretch, 155, **155**

O

Obesity, 196
Oblique exercises
   alternating twisting crunch, 132, **132**, **176**
   torso twist, 133, **133**, **184**
Oblique stretches
   cobra rising, 162, **162**
   standing torso twist, 162, **162**
One-legged lunge, for toning lower body, 88, **88**, **183**
Open arms, for stretching arms, 157, **157**
Opposite arm and leg raise, for toning full body, 52, **52**, **176**
Osteoporosis, preventing, 9
Overhead reach, for stretching shoulders, 156, **156**

P

Partner ball toss, for toning abdominals, 131, **131**, **188**
Pedaling, in bicycling, 209
Plateau
   in strength training, 177–78
   program for overcoming, 178–80, **179–80**
   weight-loss, 200
PlateMates, 36
Power walking, 220–23
Power yoga. *See* Astanga yoga
Praise pose, for stretching shoulders, 156, **156**
Prayer, during exercise, 251

Programs
   advanced, 181–84, **183–84**
   beginner
      starting, 171–72
      weeks 1 through 4 of, 173, **173**
      weeks 5 through 8 of, 174, **174**
      weeks 9 through 12 of, 175, **175**
      weeks 13 through 16 of, 176, **176**
   guidelines for selecting, 169–70
   intermediate, 177–80, **179–80**
   lower body–intensive, 185–88, **187–88**
   self-designed
      sample journal page for, **191**
      selecting exercises for, 189–90, 190
Protein, in eating plan, 257–58
Pullup, for toning upper body, 79, **79**, **183**
Punch, in martial arts aerobics, 205
Pushup, for toning upper body, 70, **70**, **176**, **183**, **188**
Pushup test, for upper-body strength, 245, 245
Pyramid sets, 18

Q

Quadriceps exercises
   leg extension, 115, **115**, **176**
   seated straight-leg lift, 114, **114**, **173**

Quadriceps stretches
  bench stretch, 163, **163**
  stork stretch, 163, **163**

R

Rate of perceived exertion, for
    aerobic exercise, <u>198</u>
Rectus abdominis exercises
  chair curl, 127, **127**, **174**
  hand-to-foot ball curl, 130,
    130, **180**
  in and out, 129, **129**, **179**,
    184
  partner ball toss, 131, **131**
  reverse curl, 128, **128**,
    175
  2-second floor crunch, 126,
    126, **173**
Repair kit, bicycling, 208
Repetitions, in strength training,
    17
Resistance bands, 26–29, 190
Rest, after strength training,
    18–19
Reverse curl, for toning
    abdominals, 128, **128**,
    175
Reverse extension, for toning
    back, 143, **143**, **184**
Reverse grip row, for toning
    back, 142, **142**, **183**
Rewards, as motivation, <u>272</u>
Rising and setting sun, for
    toning full body, 56, **56**,
    179, **188**
Road bikes, 207
Rock climbing trips, 264–65
Rockette, for toning lower body,
    85, **85**, **180**
Rope jumping, 239–41

Row and kickback, for toning
    upper body, 76, **76**,
    176
Rubber band sidestep, for
    toning butt, 109, **109**,
    180, **187**
Running, 210–13, 220
Running the rack, 18

S

Saddle bag, for bicycling, 208
Sea kayaking trips, 265
Seated back fly, for toning upper
    body, 68, **68**, **173**
Seated inner-leg lift, for toning
    inner thighs, 120, **120**,
    176
Seated row, for toning upper
    body, 74, **74**, **175**, **188**
Seated straight-leg lift, for
    toning quadriceps, 114,
    114, **173**, **188**
Self-designed programs
  sample journal page for, **191**
  selecting exercises for,
    189–90, <u>190</u>
Self-hug, for stretching upper
    back, 159, **159**
Sets
  recommended number of, 17
  types of, 17–18
Sexiness, from exercise 250
Shampoo, for swimmers, 232
Shoes
  for astanga yoga, 218
  for elliptical training, 229
  for martial arts aerobics,
    203
  for power walking, 220–21
  for rope jumping, 240

for running, 211
for snowshoeing, 237
for strength training, 12–13
for world-dance aerobics,
    225
Shorts, bicycling, 208
Shoulder exercises
  front arm raise, 97, **97**
  lateral lift, 96, **96**, **175**
  water pitcher fly, 98, **98**,
    180
Shoulder stretches
  overhead reach, 156, **156**
  praise pose, 156, **156**
Side kick, in martial arts
    aerobics, <u>205</u>
Side-lying side kick, for toning
    butt, 105, **105**, **175**,
    187
Side step and squat, for toning
    lower body, 87, **87**,
    184
Side to side, for toning lower
    body, 82, **82**, **174**
Side-to-side stretch, for
    stretching neck, 155,
    155
Simultaneous dumbbell curl, for
    toning biceps, 91, **91**,
    173
Single-arm crossover, for toning
    chest, 148, **148**, **180**,
    187
Sit and reach, for stretching
    hamstrings, 164, **164**
Skin-fold test, for measuring
    body composition, 243
Smoking cessation, aerobic
    exercise and, 198
Snacks, in eating plan, 261
Snowshoeing, 236–38
Snowshoes
  selecting, 236, 237
  technique for using, 238